Time Was

Time Was

RICHARD

BERCZELLER

THE VIKING PRESS

New York

First published in 1971 by The Viking Press, Inc.
625 Madison Avenue, New York, N.Y. 10022

Published simultaneously in Canada by
The Macmillan Company of Canada Limited

SBN 670–71563–8

Library of Congress catalog card number: 75–132859

Printed in U.S.A. by H. Wolff Book Mfg. Co.

Parts of this book originally appeared in
The New Yorker in somewhat different form.

To Peter Hanns

My heartfelt thanks to Rachel MacKenzie. Without her encouragement this book would never have been written.

Contents

Time Was

THE CAFÉ KLINIK . . .
AND GRETL

A certain summer day in 1920 is easy to remember now as a turning point, even though it seemed trivial then. On that day I was
listening to Kurt Lacker, the goalkeeper of the soccer team of
which I was the right wing. Kurt was a third-year medical student, and I was to enter medical school in the fall. Kurt spoke
about medical school, and the professors and the dissecting room
and other odds and ends, but chiefly he spoke about the Café
Klinik. The Café Klinik was located at the very center of Vienna
and seemed to be at least as important as anatomy or pathology.
With wide gestures Kurt described it. "An extraordinary place,"
he said. "Terrific! One of the great cafés of Vienna. The very best
coffee, a fluffy Gugelhupf. And the service! Herr Franz, the Ober,
may look a little reserved, standoffish, you know, but he has a
heart of gold, with a particularly soft spot for medical students.
He will even borrow money for you."

"You mean," I said, "he will lend you money."

"No. I mean what I said—he will borrow from the other patrons to lend to you, if he likes you. The most important thing for
you to remember, Richard, as you enter Vienna, is Herr Franz."

At that time we were living in Baden bei Wien, only half an hour from Vienna. We were refugees from fascist Hungary; Father was barely making a living, and the financial basis on which I was to start my medical studies seemed perilously frail—shaky, rather. A relative of ours in Vienna had offered a couch in his living room for sleeping purposes, and I could go home for weekends. Perhaps everything would work out.

Winter begins early in that part of the world, and the usual icy wind blew from the nearby Alps. Mother accompanied me to the railroad station on September 21. She talked about the traffic in Vienna. "Look left, look right, then look again." She had packed my suitcase—all clean clothes, freshly washed and ironed, and groceries: a loaf of bread, a large piece of salami, and Mohnstrudel, my favorite dessert. "Your studies are important," she said, "but health comes first. Be sure to look after your feet. A doctor spends much of his life on his feet." She mentioned traffic again and kissed me.

As I entered Vienna I thought of Herr Franz and the Café Klinik, and so, even before going to my relatives, I took a trolley to the medical-school district. The famous establishment was not where Kurt had said it would be—but then I looked again and saw it; the sign said it was: a tiny café with a couple of tables outdoors. I went in and smelled coffee and dust and tobacco, and saw a cleaning woman mopping the floor in the light of an unshaded bulb. A short heavy figure came toward me, and I knew, I sensed, that this was Herr Franz. He had a bald head, small eyes, a mustache.

"The café is closed," he said. "We don't open until seventhirty."

"Are you Herr Franz?" I asked.

"Well?"

"I'm a first-year medical-school student," I said. "A friend told me about you. I'm sorry. I'll come back later."

"*Das ist was anderes,*" Herr Franz said. "Sit down." With a commanding gesture he told the cleaning woman to take the chairs off the nearest table. "What will you have?" he asked.

"A cup of coffee, Herr Franz."

He came back from the kitchen with a cup of coffee and also a piece of Gugelhupf. "You must be hungry. Eat. Where did you say you came from?"

I told him.

"Yes, yes," he said. "I was there during the war, at the Café Central on the Hauptplatz. I waited even on the Kaiser. What newspaper do you want?" A Viennese café without newspapers does not exist.

"The *Neue Freie Presse,* Herr Franz."

"Good," he said and brought me the *Neue Freie Presse.*

I drank my coffee and ate my cake and read the news. Amundsen's Arctic expedition was still in trouble; his ship, the *Maud,* was stuck in the ice off the Siberian coast. Dispatch from Berlin: The Red Army, led by General Budënny, had been thrashed and routed by the Poles. The mayor of Cork, Ireland, was continuing his hunger strike. The majority of a congress of physicists at Bad Nauheim, Germany, discussing Einstein's theory of relativity, doubted its value. A new film directed by Ernst Lubitsch starred an actress named Pola Negri, who gave a brilliant performance.

Someone wearing pince-nez was peering over my shoulder. He took off the pince-nez and became Herr Franz. "Amundsen," he said, "a stupid man, going the wrong way. He should have started from the other side—Greenland. It is only necessary to look at the map to realize that. As far as Einstein and his theory are concerned, I've been thinking it over and it is hardly believable. The poor mayor of Cork—another stupid man. Why did he trust the British? The British are no good, never have been." He put on the pince-nez and looked at the paper again. "Pola Negri," he said. "And what is so special about her? She rolls her eyes and moves her ass. A woman, like them all."

Other patrons of the Café Klinik began to arrive, young men with books under their arms. Herr Franz addressed each one by his name. I was sure he had forgotten me, but presently he returned.

"The first thing you need is a room," he said.

I told him about my relative and the couch in the living room. "Bah," he said. "Relatives are no good when you are young. They are always saying, 'Come home early, no smoking, no singing.' And it is not *Sturmfrei*. You are a grown man, aren't you? You don't have the look of a virgin." He blinked.

Herr Franz was right. Where would I take a girl? Herr Franz took a notebook from his pocket and turned the pages. "Yes," he said, "here is an address: Frau Tesarek, Parhammerplatz Twelve. Her husband died in nineteen-sixteen, the last Brusilov offensive. A pretty little woman, young, living off the few crowns she gets as her widow's pension. Only ten minutes by trolley. Try it."

"I will, Herr Franz."

He put the book away. "For any problems come to me."

The Parhammerplatz was in the Hernals district—one- or two-story houses, here and there a sprinkling of little parks. At Number 12 I walked up one flight and found the name of the late Herr Tesarek on the door. I rang the bell, and someone called, "Who is it?"

"Herr Franz of the Café Klinik sent me," I replied.

The door opened.

"Frau Tesarek?"

"Yes," she said. "Come in."

I was astonished. Herr Franz had said, "A pretty little woman, young." Pretty? Her eyes weren't bad, and she had good teeth, but such a thin face! And she was getting on—twenty-eight at least, perhaps even thirty.

She showed me around her apartment: one room and a kitchen. "But where is the room for rent?" I asked.

"This," she said.

"But then, Frau Tesarek, what about you?"

"Oh, I sleep in the kitchen. Do you like the room? Please take it. You don't have to pay in advance." She wiped her hands on her sky-blue apron, which was spotlessly clean. There were two windows in the room, and the inevitable geranium pots, a table, two chairs, a large bed with lots of quilts, but no electric light. "Kerosene lamp only," Frau Tesarek explained. "It makes nice light."

"All right, Frau Tesarek."

A man in uniform, with a heavy mustache, stared at me from the wall. Frau Tesarek followed my eyes. "I will take him down, if he disturbs you, but—I would like him to stay here, not in the kitchen, if you don't mind."

"I don't mind, Frau Tesarek."

"Thank you," she said. "He was a good man. Would you care for a cup of coffee?"

Physics, biology, chemistry, anatomy, histology, physiology—six hours of lectures every day, plus the laboratories. I can hear the voices in each lecture room. "Anatomy is the backbone of medicine!" exclaimed Professor Tandler enthusiastically. "Biology— the backbone of medicine," said soft-spoken Professor Wittmann. "Could medicine even be thought of without a knowledge of physics?" asked Professor Lecher, waggling his Santa Claus beard. Professor Fromm, chemistry, limped around his lab (his right leg had been amputated after the battle of the Isonzo River) and pointed toward the General Hospital. "Those famous clinicians," he said with heavy irony, "could they treat their patients without remembering just a bit of chemistry?" And Professor Schaffer, histology, thundered from his beard, "The microscope opened a new world! Without it where would we be? From the microscope came light, light, light!"

But we freshmen were most impressed by anatomy. In the amphitheater we looked down at a table where human bones were displayed. Professor Tandler, a stocky man with a huge mustache, explained that the prominences had once held tendons, and in these narrow channels blood vessels and nerves had fulfilled their functions. Each bone (the body seemed to be made up of a countless number) had its name. The tiny bones of the wrist: os naviculare, lunatum, triquetrum, pisiform, multangulum majus and minus, capitatum, hamatum—I have not forgotten them. Only after learning the name and purpose of every bone could one enter the dissecting laboratory.

It was a strange feeling to touch a dead body for the first time. Here was the supreme test of whether the medical student would be able to stand the strain of the profession. The first sight of the corpses on the dissecting tables did not encourage youngsters with weak nerves. Most of us were pale and quiet, quiet as death, when we entered those vast gloomy chambers and sniffed the strange smell in the air—alcohol and formalin, to prevent decomposition. Some keeled over and were carried out, perhaps to try again, perhaps not. My friend Kurt the goalkeeper (sitting on the soccer ball, as all goalkeepers do) had warned me, and I had wondered: was I to be one of the weaklings? No, but even now, half a century later, I still have that feeling of nausea and fear—and also of pride. Here I was, eighteen, only yesterday a boy in the Gymnasium, reading the unforgettable words above the professor's podium:

HIC LOCUS EST UBI MORS GAUDET SUCCURERE VITAE
(*Here death is happy to help the living*)

Tandler, unforgettable Tandler! He always seemed to have a cigar in his mouth. I was dissecting on a female pelvis when the cigar smell came through the formalin smell and I found Tandler looking over my shoulder. In silence he watched; in silence I worked, as diligently as I could, waiting for the question. Once, the story ran, he asked a student, "How long is the conjugata

vera?" Normally the conjugata vera is from ten to twelve centi-
meters, reaching from the pubic bone to the sacral bone, an important indication of the size of the female pelvis, which carries
the baby. The nervous young man replied, "Twenty-five centime-
ters, Herr Professor." "With a conjugata vera that size," Tandler
remarked, "the baby could run around in it and even rest com-
fortably on a chamber pot." By and by the cigar smell went away
as Tandler moved to another table.

A Social Democrat, he was Health and Hospital Commissioner
of the City of Vienna. Vienna had just begun to recover from the
misery of the war's aftermath; once the capital of a common-
wealth of nations numbering more than fifty million people, it
had seen Austria shrink to a little country of barely seven million.
Hunger, starvation, was everywhere, and the mortality among
children was enormous. Tandler preached, "No charity! Collective responsibility!" It was he who originated the so-called baby
packages, complete outfits of all the indispensables for the newborn. These packages went to every mother, the poor and the in-
between and the rich. That was Tandler's point. "We're not going to discriminate against the poor," he said, "even if the
wealthy get what they don't need."

He made the Hospital of the City of Vienna into the best and
most progressive in the country. At sixty-six, he was asked by the
Soviet Union to reorganize its public-health structure. He died in
Moscow in 1936; his ashes rest in Vienna.

The money Mother had given me was coming to an end. I had
to find a part-time job. As things were, I could never have got
through the mornings without the breakfast served free by the
American Quakers at the aula of the university—a large bowl of
hot chocolate and a thick slice of bread, given to you by those
good ladies with a smile and a few kind words (in an atrocious
accent). For dinner I went to the cafeteria set up by the Jewish
Joint Distribution Committee in a dilapidated building on the

Zimmermannplatz. Hundreds of young men—there weren't many women students at that time—sat around the rough wooden tables. The price of the meal was very low, and if you couldn't pay you weren't asked for it twice. In a corner was a big blackboard with lost-and-found and help-wanted notices. One day I saw this:

WANTED, A STUDENT AS FRENCH TUTOR FOR TWO CHILDREN, A BOY OF NINE, A GIRL OF EIGHT.

The address was a good one, in the fashionable Hietzing, the *Villaviertel* (upper-middle-class quarter) of Vienna; and in addition to the fee, the tutor would receive a *Jause*—afternoon coffee with coffee cake. I had never thought of myself as a French tutor, but I had had five years of French, and the thought of the *Jause* was irresistible. I hurried off to Hietzing, hoping that no other hopeful French tutors had got there first.

Herr and Frau Stieglbauer received me warmly. Alas, Herr Stieglbauer said, neither of them could speak French. I endeavored to suppress my joy at this news; no one would be in a position to judge *my* French. And the children were, thank God, delightful. I taught them the language of Molière and learned it better myself, and the *Jause* was superb.

So the immediate future seemed fairly secure: breakfast with the Quakers, dinner at the Joint Distribution Committee Cafeteria, *Jause* with the Stiegelbauers; and, thanks to that generous and friendly couple, some money in my pocket. Herr Franz looked at me with astonishment and pleasure when, one evening at the Café Klinik, I ordered two poached eggs—a great luxury—and paid for them at once, in cash.

"How are you progressing with your studies?" he asked. I told him I was progressing well. *"Gut, gut,"* he murmured and brought the eggs.

I diligently attended all the lectures. The physics hour was a pleasant interlude after the exciting anatomy lecture. I sat in the last row, and soon a comfortable feeling of somnolence would steal over me. Professor Lecher's voice, warm but weak, was hardly audible in the seclusion of my row, and as often as not I dozed off. Lecher was known all over the world for the machines he had invented, mostly generators, but I could never understand why his subject was important for the study of medicine. I would have completely forgotten about physics, I think, if it hadn't been for an episode I witnessed in his class.

At that time the papers were full of recent developments in the transmission of sound by radio. Professor Lecher explained the principles of the phenomenon with drawings and equations on the blackboard. One day he brought a strange apparatus to the classroom and announced that at twelve noon exactly we would hear twelve chimes, and the sound of the chimes would have come all the way from Big Ben *in London!* In breathless silence we watched the minute hand of the clock on the wall creep toward twelve, and exactly on the second of the minute, lo and behold, we heard the chimes—but they came from the Votivkirche in Vienna. Lecher's wireless set was mute. Nothing from London. I felt embarrassed for him, a worried-looking Santa Claus. "I'm sorry," he murmured. "Maybe next time."

Something else happened about that time. I got back to Frau Tesarek's at about eleven every night; ordinarily she wouldn't be there—visiting friends, she would explain the next morning. One evening I had been studying at the Café Klinik, chatting occasionally with Herr Franz, and missed the last trolley, which left at quarter to eleven, and so I had to walk home, which took almost an hour. I climbed the steps, carefully unlocked the kitchen door so as not to awaken Frau Tesarek, and crossed the dark kitchen on tiptoe. Ahead of me I saw a crack of light underneath my door. I slowly opened the door. Frau Tesarek was lying in my bed. The wick of the kerosene lamp was turned low, but her eyes had a greenish glint which pierced the half-darkness. Her hair, usually pinned up, was hanging loose over her bare shoulders, and the quilt did not quite come up to her breasts, which were strong, well rounded.

I stood there as though struck by lightning. She looked at me with her greenish glint and finally spoke. "What are you waiting for?" she said.

Well, what *was* I waiting for?

From then on I had plenty to eat. At night Gretl (Frau Tesarek had become Gretl) would have a snack waiting, frankfurters and a piece of chicken, cake, and real coffee. She would bring these delicacies to my room on a tray and put the tray on the bed, and we would eat, side by side, before we went to bed. Yet I didn't gain weight. One day when I came to the Café Klinik I found my mother involved in a conversation with Herr Franz (of course I had told her and father about him on my weekend visits home, which had become infrequent). "He is all right, Frau Berczeller," I heard Herr Franz say. "But does he eat enough?" she asked anxiously. "Well, he's thin," Herr Franz admitted, "but as far as I can see he's not starving. *Da kann ma halt nix machen.* It's nature. Also, he has been—" He saw me and chuckled.

Occasionally I didn't hear the alarm clock and would be too late for the anatomy lecture, which I couldn't afford to miss. Gretl took over. The alarm never rang in vain. Women, I discovered at that time, have a keener sense of hearing.

During the fall months of 1920 I studied chemistry, histology, and physiology. Fromm, our chemistry professor, was internationally known; immediately following the war his name was almost constantly in the news. He had been one of the heads of the poison-gas team of the German Army, a group of scientists who had developed that deadly weapon. It was tried out against the French and Canadians, and they, unprepared for the assault, died by the tens of thousands, until the gas mask, developed with frantic haste, put a stop to the slaughter. Fromm's name had a prominent place on the list of war criminals presented by the Allies to the German and Austrian governments. The demand for their punishment was never honored; the Kaiser had fled to Holland, and in Germany itself many of the generals on the list were back in positions of power. Fromm himself received the much coveted appointment at Vienna University. (Even if he had been handed over to the Allies, it is likely that he would have prospered, just as his successors, the German scientists of the Second World War, were welcomed with open arms by the United States, Britain, and the Soviet Union.)

Fromm was a great teacher. Limping around among the Bunsen burners, he spoke eloquently on his subject, and also on political matters. The legend of the *Dolchstoss von hinten,* the stab in the back, first reached me all mixed up with potassium and magnesium. "Our troops were victorious on all fronts," Fromm said. "Victory was within reach. But in the *Hinterland* a treacherous group of agitators grasped the evil blade and struck."

I couldn't stand this without saying something. "My father was in the war, Herr Professor," I said. "He was missing in action, and for months we thought he was dead. When he finally came home he was thin and weak, with scars from his terrible grenade wounds. And as for those of us at home—well, we had hardly anything to eat."

"The soldier's duty is to die for the Fatherland, young man!" Fromm thundered. "The Socialists and Jews—" His expression spoke for him.

But he had a sense of humor. He remembered the episode but gave me an A in chemistry all the same. "You would have made a good soldier," he said. "Brave, courageous, although a bit impudent. You aren't Jewish by any chance?"

"I am."

"Hmm," he said, looking embarrassed. "Let me tell you a story one of my colleagues at the Army research laboratories told me. A poor man went to his tailor to have his torn jacket repaired, and the tailor said the jacket would be ready in a few days. It wasn't. Altogether it took thirty days. When the man finally got it back he said, 'You've taken thirty days to mend my jacket, and God only needed seven to make the world!' 'Look at the beautiful job I've done on your jacket,' said the tailor. 'Then take a look at the world.' "

Fromm looked up from behind his glasses and gave me a pat on the shoulder. "My colleague is Jewish," he remarked. "Excellent anecdotes."

Histology: I still feel butterflies in my stomach when I think of the somber Institute of Histology building. Professor Schaffer's monotonous voice practically invited his students to take a nap. The only time his voice rose above its dull drone was when he had occasion to speak of his predecessor, Victor Ritter von Rofenstein, who had started the research in the growth of bone tissue, spermatogenesis. In the histology lab we bent over the microscope, learning how to handle it. It seemed to be an impossible undertaking even to reflect light from the source, a candle; but little by little I learned how to differentiate the tissues of the various parts of the body by deciphering the tiny elements of which they were composed. Certainly I never had the talent to become one of the great histologists; I ask myself what I would do now, after forty-four years in practice, if I had to make a microscopic differentiation of the pancreas, the kidney, the intestine, a blood vessel.

After the physics exam, half a dozen of us who had passed it had a victory celebration at the Café Klinik. Herr Franz, always precisely informed about all medical students' events, was waiting with a *Stamperl* of Cognac for each of us. The party went on much longer than we'd thought it would, which is usually true of medical students' celebrations; others had joined in, many with their girls. The billiard table (that indispensable item of all

Viennese cafés) was pushed into a corner, somebody struck up on his violin, and there was dancing and singing. I had a bag with me containing two bottles of Gumpoldskirchner, a strong dry white wine made from grapes grown on the sandy hillsides near Vienna, a Torte, and a can of sardines—not for the chemistry-exam celebration but for a surprise party for Gretl.

At quarter to eleven I left the celebration—reluctantly, but I wanted to get home in plenty of time to fix up the kitchen table in really festive style. Gretl wouldn't believe her eyes. She seldom came home before eleven, so I walked through the unusually warm night rather than catching the last trolley. *"Jessas Maria!"* Gretl would exclaim when she saw the feast.

I walked toward the Gürtel, the boulevard separating Vienna from the outskirts. Soon I heard a woman's voice: *"Bubi,* how about coming with me?" The Gürtel was known as the Boulevard of the Whores, so this was no surprise; it had happened often before. I would politely decline the invitation, and then the girl would say, *"Schade.* You have such a kind voice. Maybe ten schillings is too much? Why don't we talk it over?" The street lights in postwar Vienna were a good five hundred meters from one another, and most of the Gürtel was in semi-darkness.

The voice again: *"Bubi,* what about it?" The girl took my arm, and I became aware of her perfume. It was intensely familiar, as it should have been, a violet perfume I'd bought only a few weeks ago. I didn't say anything; I couldn't seem to think, but walked on numbly until we came to the next street light, and then I saw her: Gretl. How ugly she was, with her hair piled high on her head and her cheeks ridiculously rouged!

"There is a nice hotel close by," she murmured in the motherly voice I knew so well. She really looked at me for the first time. She gave a little cry. I walked quickly away, in the direction of the Parhammerplatz.

I smelled the violets again as she came running after me. She didn't speak, and I didn't. Suddenly I became aware of the bag under my arm—the wine, the Torte, the sardines. In a sudden rage I threw it down: bang!

Gretl's tearful voice: "But how else could I have got the money for the frankfurters, the chicken, the coffee?"

I walked on; she followed. We came to the house. I ran up the steps, opened the door, lit the kerosene lamp, turned the wick high, took down my rucksack and suitcase.

All my clothes had been neatly arranged by Gretl. As I left I heard her muffled cries.

I spent the night on a park bench. It was a beautiful night, the kind of night, I used to think, that you could find only in Vienna. I hadn't really been in love with Gretl; she was more like a sister or a mother, a warm, secure place, and I had always been impatient to see her at night, to see her shadow with its full contours on the wall when she brought in the tray and put it on the bed. She wasn't the first lover I had had. A little housemaid had seduced me when I was fifteen, and then in Baden bei Wien, I used to go to the Kurpark with an enthusiastic soccer fan, a girl of sixteen with fiery hair. Far back in the park, where it was dark and the meadow grass was soft and sweet, we made love while she babbled on about soccer and what a terrific right wing I was.

Very stiff and sore, I got up off the park bench in the morning and walked to the trolley station. What should I do now? The answer was clear: go to the Café Klinik.

Herr Franz listened intently. I was amazed when his face, always immaculately shaved in the morning, broke into a wide smile. "I can only tell you an anecdote about one of your countrymen, Ferenc Molnár," he began. "I heard it when I was a waiter at the officers' club during the war. Molnár had a beautiful girl friend in Budapest. He was at the height of his fame and traveled all over Europe, wherever his plays were produced, but always, faithfully, at the beginning of every month he sent his little friend a check. Once when he got back to Budapest he heard a rumor: she had cheated on him, not once or twice but with lots of men. Molnár listened to the shocking story and pressed that famous monocle of his deeper into the furrow around his right eye. 'Well, there's still a difference between all her beaux and me,' he observed. 'I'm the only one who *pays* her.' In your case," Herr Franz concluded, "it's exactly the opposite, *nicht wahr?*"

{ ii }

THE STANDEE WITH
THE ASH-BLOND HAIR

In bleak postwar Vienna, music was a ray of hope for a brighter future. There were fears that the once-proud city would not be able to keep her traditional role as a world center of the arts, music especially, but the fears came to nothing. In the unheated Opera House and concert halls the musicians played with freezing fingers. The audience sat bundled up in winter clothes, watching the singers in flimsy costumes on the stage. The quality of the productions was as good as ever, perhaps even better, despite the arctic air. There were premières: on October 1, 1919, Richard Strauss's *Die Frau ohne Schatten* with Maria Jeritza as the Empress and Lotte Lehmann as the Dyer's Wife. I was seventeen then. The second time I heard it was at the Metropolitan Opera House in New York, fifty years later.

Guest performers had often come to my home town in Hungary, Sopron (Ödenburg), from Vienna, which was only seventy kilometers away. In our ancient "burgher town" music belonged to the *guter Ton*. I was taken to concerts by Grandmother, later by Mother; Father had a deaf ear for music and heard nothing when I went around the house whistling Puccini and Verdi arias.

I first heard the *Pastorale* and the Ninth Symphony in our *Kaszinó,* also Bruckner's Eighth, which I was not to hear again until 1967, with Herbert von Karajan conducting at Carnegie Hall.

And so it was only natural that one of the first things I did when I came to Vienna to enter medical school was to go to the opera, a performance of *Rigoletto.* With many other young people I watched from the standing room of the fourth gallery. Many of them were Conservatory students who followed the score as they listened. We were packed in pretty closely. One of my nearest neighbors was a girl of seventeen or so with ash-blond hair hanging down to her shoulders, and a daintily pointed nose. She had eyes for nothing but her score. Occasionally she dropped a page, and I picked it up and gave it back to her. She did not glance at me, just murmured, *"Danke schön."*

Standing room was cheap, and I went to the opera often. The girl with the ash-blond hair was always there, leaning against one of the pillars. Once, on October 10, I saw her at the Konzerthaussaal. I remember the date because it was the 150th anniversary of Beethoven's birth, celebrated with the Leonore Overture Number 3 and the Ninth Symphony. We didn't seem to take to each other. She was a pretty girl; so were many girls in Vienna.

The Gretl episode ended. I was depressed. The opera was my only consolation (except for Herr Franz). I saw my first performance of *Tosca,* with Jeritza in the title role, Piccaver as Cavaradossi, and, if I remember correctly, Jerger as Scarpia—a brilliant performance. The last act: the firing squad, commanded by the evil Spoletta, fires, and the mortally wounded Cavaradossi falls. Tosca discovers the treachery of Scarpia, whom she murdered after he had falsely promised to spare her beloved's life. "Mario!" she screams. "Mario, Mario, Mario!" Led by Spoletta, the firing squad reappears; the dead Scarpia has been found, and they have come to arrest Tosca. She runs to the parapet overlooking Rome and jumps into the yawning abyss—a typical heroic end for *die* Jeritza, tall, magnificent, her reddish-blond hair disheveled, a gesture of vigor and desperation. While the curtain quickly fell, the orchestra played *"E lucevan le stelle . . ."*

Deeply moved, the audience sat in silence; then came a storm of applause. A thought entered my mind, and I laughed.

"Barbarian!" someone said. I turned and saw the ash-blond girl. She looked at me with contempt.

"I—I'm sorry," I stammered. "Please let me explain."

"Barbarian," she said again and pursed her lips. She collected her music and with a haughty glance pushed past me.

I was furious and embarrassed. Others had heard me laugh, and they too were looking at me as if I were a barbarian. I hurried out.

At the trolley station, I saw the ash-blond girl. It had started to rain. I had a coat; she didn't. "Will you take my coat, Fräulein?" I said.

"No!" she snapped.

Then I really lost my temper. "I don't give a damn what you think of me," I said, "but I can only tell you you're a snob."

"What?"

I looked into deer-brown eyes with wide pupils. "Now listen," I said, "I want to tell you something. Then you can go your way and I'll go mine. I laughed back there because of something my grandmother told me when I was a little boy. A provincial opera company had come to our town. They performed *Tosca*. The last act: The parapet; Tosca jumps, *and*—"

I paused and looked deep into the deer-brown eyes.

"A moment later Spoletta runs to the parapet and somersaults over."

"What?" she said again but with quite a different inflection. *"He* jumped *too?"*

"Yes," I said. "The curtain got stuck."

She stared at me until she understood, then burst into laughter. "That's the funniest thing I've ever heard. Tomorrow I'll tell it all around the Conservatory."

Her trolley arrived. She boarded it and waved from the platform. "You're *not* a barbarian," she shouted.

I had to find another room, but Herr Franz couldn't help me; it was only a short time before vacation, and nothing was available. I spent the remaining month on the living-room couch of our relative. How right Herr Franz was! I had to be home on time. I was steadily asked questions.

The Stieglbauer job came to an end for the time being. I studied more diligently than ever, went more often to the physiology lectures late in the afternoon. Professor Durig was a debonair man who wore a sports suit, quite unlike the other professors, who were always in formal clothes. With close attention I listened to him lecture on the circulation of the blood, the function of different organs, heat-regulation.

I spent the three vacation months with my parents. The Badener Athletic Club received me with open arms, and so did the soccer-loving girl friend. Of course I intended to study; alas, my books rested peacefully in the suitcase. I had already passed the physics, biology, and chemistry exams, but anatomy, physiology, and the rest of the basic sciences still lay ahead. Every night I went to bed vowing that the next morning would be devoted to study, and fell asleep with the pleasant feeling of good intentions. I would get up at eleven, go for a swim, and then settle on a hill in a quiet corner of the Kurpark with the anatomy atlas. That was what I told myself. Of course on my way there I'd run into one of my friends and all study plans would dissipate.

The two years I had lived in Baden with my family were the last part of my early youth. The town's history went back to the Romans, who had discovered the healing properties of the sulphur baths. Now the population was around twenty-two thousand; the buildings were mostly Biedermeier, with additions of rococo and the tasteless architecture of the nouveaux-riches who had their summer homes in the neighborhood of the old aristocracy. In the kiosk of the Kurpark the band played twice daily (on rainy days in the Kurhaus), and the latest operettas could be seen in the small baroque theater near the main square. You could guess that some of the men passing by had been imperial officers, because they straightened and touched their fingers to their hats when they passed the building on the Hauptplatz which had been the headquarters of His Imperial Majesty, who was now in exile far away.

Neither the martial reputation of the town nor the healing properties of the spa had brought my family to Baden bei Wien. After we fled the White Terror of the Horthy government in Hungary, an old uncle, a Jewish butcher, invited us to Baden. For us he was a life-saver. In a time of food rationing so severe that it was only a little better than starving to death, the butcher and baker became all-powerful. I can still taste beef drippings whenever I think of Baden. Uncle brought home an indispensable plate of fat hidden under his blood-sprinkled apron. He was a very small man, almost a dwarf, taciturn but with lively little eyes that twinkled when he reached under his apron and presented Mother with a fresh plate of drippings.

Beef dripping is hard to digest; it solidifies when only slightly below boiling temperature, then settles to the bottom of a pan like dirty snow. It filled the stomach and tasted like candles. As soon as Mother brought it to the table we devoured it—but not all; some was saved for bartering purposes with people who had a baker uncle.

When I think of Baden I also smell the sulphur fumes from the pores of the earth. Residents of the town were permitted to use the baths without charge. We youngsters used them as swimming pools, liberally, also as rendezvous, because both sexes were allowed in at the same time. Those who came in search of healing were pushed to the periphery.

City ordinances proclaimed that the spas were strictly for therapeutic purposes, and the aged warden cautioned us again and

again, without effect. Finally two policemen appeared, elderly
men with big mustaches. We greeted them with splashes and soon
had them drenched and smelling to high heaven of sulphur. Next
came the Mayor. He was the wealthiest haberdasher in town
(later he became a cabinet minister). We greeted him respectfully, with no splashing. *"Guten Tag, Herr Bürgermeister,"* we
said and stood at attention.

Pleased, he nodded. "What do you want?" he said sharply to
the trembling warden. "They behave as if they're in kindergar-
ten."

The leaves of the tall linden trees turned yellow and brown,
and wrinkled and fell, and September was here, time to go back
to Vienna.

Herr Franz took out his little booklet and ran through the ad-
dresses. They were all too expensive for my very meager budget,
because unfortunately the Stieglbauer job was gone for good.
With tears, Frau Stieglbauer told me that her husband's business
had deteriorated to such a degree that they had had to let their
chauffeur go, also their two maids and the *Kinderfräulein;* they
certainly could not afford a French tutor. *"Au revoir, cher Mon-
sieur,"* the two children said sadly.

I heard about a Socialist student home maintained by the
Union Council. As a Socialist, at any rate the son of a Socialist
father, I was accepted. There were two large dormitories resembling army barracks, with thirty iron cots in each. As long as the
mild autumn weather lasted, the home was bearable, but then
winter came down like a wolf; that winter of 1921–1922 still
makes me shiver. There was no fuel in the student home, the
little stove in the corner was cold as ice; but one was young and
soon warmed up under the two thin blankets. The Quaker breakfast brought back life and hope.

Now there could be no excuses for not studying. A difficult semester lay ahead: anatomy, histology, and physiology. At night I

studied exclusively at the Café Klinik. The student home was within walking distance.

My way to medical school led me through the Berggasse, where I almost always saw an elderly gentleman with a gray beard, hands clasped behind him, leaving his house. He was Professor Freud (during my student years he did not lecture at the medical school). His eyes would turn rather absently toward me, I would greet him with respect, and he would murmur "*Guten Morgen.*" There was always the same exchange, but I don't think he ever recognized me.

I always looked out for the ash-blond girl at the opera, but I didn't see her again until late autumn. There she was, leaning against the pillar, studying her score (I think the opera was Richard Strauss's *Salomé*). Standing room was jammed, as always. I waited for her to raise her eyes. At last she did, and saw me. She smiled and gestured, and I pushed my way through the crowd to her side. "Spoletta," she whispered, giggling.

Afterward I asked her to have a cup of coffee with me at the Opern Café, an artists' rendezvous nearby. As we came in she drew my attention to someone sitting at a window table, the composer Alban Berg (very few people knew him then; his *Wozzeck* was not produced until 1930). She couldn't stay very long, she said as we sat down, because she had to be home by eleven at the latest, and it was a half-hour trip by trolley to where she lived with an old uncle.

"Where is that?" I asked.

"Near Schönbrunn," she told me. She wasn't quite as pretty as I'd thought at first; she had a very pale complexion, and her lower lip protruded slightly. We had a pleasant if rather academic talk. She spoke about music, and I explained some of the pictures in my anatomy atlas, which always faithfully accompanied me. We made a date to meet again at the opera in a week.

The weather grew worse; so did my financial resources—it is a grotesque exaggeration to call them resources. A struggling film company paid five schillings a day for extras, but this income came to an end with winter. And Father was out of work. I gave German lessons to a Hungarian newspaperman. Hungarians are proverbially generous, but when it came to paying for the lessons Gerényi *úr* behaved as though he hadn't heard; he was far less generous than the Stieglbauers had been for their children's French lessons (once I saw poor Stieglbauer peddling stationery in a small café).

I managed, though, to go on paying for standing room and to take the very pale ash-blond girl to the Opern Café afterward. Our conversation stayed academic, but I learned her name and began to call her Liesl. "My father insists on my being called Elisabeth," she said. Her second name was—let us say—Hohengraben. I asked her if she was related to the former chief of staff on the Russian front. Her pale complexion turned delicately pink. "My father," she said. She came from an old aristocratic family that had given many of its sons to the Habsburg Empire's military elite.

I went on calling her Liesl and finally managed to persuade her to call me Richard. "Now, Liesl, how do you feel sitting here with a commoner, a republican—and a Jew?" I asked one day.

"Oh, don't be absurd," she said.

A little while before Christmas she invited me to her home. By then I was deeply in love. I had even kissed her a few times.

Her uncle was a widower, and they lived in an old house which from outside looked like an abandoned rococo palace with huge neglected gardens surrounding it. Once a *Sektionschef* in the Imperial Ministry of Commerce, the old man had lost his savings in war bonds and spent his time writing his memoirs. "Poor uncle," Liesl said, "he thinks a publisher will be interested in how the *K. und K.* [*Kaiserlich und Königlich*] Ministry of Commerce was managed in 1899." A cleaning lady came once a week to tidy up—or perhaps it was every other week.

Old Eduard Ritter von Kosubski was almost completely deaf, and when Liesl introduced me she had to shout my name a few times. I shouted it in a louder voice. Finally he nodded. *"Ja, ja,"* he said in a deaf man's soft voice. "The Baron Berkovitzki, he was your uncle?"

Liesl whispered, "Say yes."

I smiled and nodded, and the old man nodded again. "It doesn't really make any difference," Liesl told me later when we were sitting together at the piano in her room, a room with a ceiling as high as that of a church. "I'd already told him you were a medical student and he wasn't too happy with the revelation. 'Be careful,' he warned me. 'We are besieged by proletarians. Think of your father, your grandfather, and your great-grandfather! Think of your ancestor Count Klingenstein, the greatest general in the Army, who captured the flag of the Grand Vizier of the Turkish army that besieged Vienna in 1683!' " Liesl stroked my cheek. "By now he's forgotten your plebeian origin," she murmured.

Those late winter afternoons in the Schönbrunnerstrasse! At four, darkness flowed slowly into the old room with baroque windows, against which icicles hung, and Liesl played. She played Chopin, Mendelssohn, Bach, Handel. Her fine childlike fingers strolled and danced and fluttered on the faintly yellowed keys, and the shadows deepened over her pale face. Several rooms away, the deaf old man wrote on and on about mighty deeds in the Ministry of Commerce. A perfume which Liesl said she had inherited from her mother was sweet and poignant in the frosty air. "Liesl," I said, "we are two grown-up people and we are in love. Should we settle just for kisses?"

"Yes," she said. "How often do I have to tell you?"

"But why?"

"Because I was told: only after marriage."

"Then I'll marry you."

She laughed. "Right here?"

"Don't make fun of me. Three or four years from now I'll be a doctor."

"My father would never give his consent."

"You don't have to ask him."

"I'm a minor."

"Let's elope."

"Richard!" she said. "Be sensible. There are your medical studies, and then also—well, there's *me*. I mean I have to get used to the idea. I know it's ridiculous and archaic, but I'm still a Hohengraben."

"You can't be serious."

"Please give me time."

Herr Franz studied me, his thin brows pulled up to his hairline. "You have lost weight," he declared. "Why? You study hard, but so does everyone here. It must be something else. A woman?"

"The most beautiful on earth."

"That," Herr Franz said, "I have already heard more than enough. Two billion women, all beautiful. Where are the ugly ones?"

"I want to marry her."

"What?" he exclaimed. "You're only in your third semester! Another five years to graduation. And then, the internship, residency. . . . How can you support a wife?"

"She plays the piano," I said, "beautifully. We will manage."

"Now listen. I don't like to interfere in anyone else's business because I don't like it if anyone interferes in mine. But love and marriage—different things, *wissens?* Love—rosy skies. Marriage? Marriage *ist eine In-sti-tu-tion*. It is like the government. It gives security—let us say a bit of security. On the other hand, you have to pay taxes to it. Taxes, taxes, taxes, until you are bled white. Understand?"

"No," I said.

"There is an old proverb," Herr Franz said, "that if the penis thinks, then common sense is in the ass. All girls carry a more or less precious heritage between their more or less well-formed legs.

It is good for us. But why want it as a monopoly? Don't marry her!"

"She doesn't want to get married." I groaned.

His eyebrows came down, and he grinned. "Lucky man! This happens only once in a million years. Congratulations."

"You see, she is a Hohengraben."

There was a short silence. "That is something else," Herr Franz said finally. "This girl is smarter than you. People of different classes shouldn't associate too much with one another. What would you do with a countess, a Catholic, as your wife? Once I saw General Rüdiger Graf von Hohengraben. Eyes like steel. Forget it!"

"I can't forget it."

"My God, how often I've heard that during these thirty-five years! And now all those lovesick young men are big professors with wives, children, grandchildren. They didn't marry the pretty little girls who made them sick with love; they married plain women of good middle-class society."

"With us it will be different," I said stubbornly.

Herr Franz made an impatient gesture, and I opened my anatomy book. He went to another table and asked for orders. I continued to read.

Suddenly I heard his voice again, whispering in my ear so that the people at the neighboring table wouldn't become interested. "Listen to reason. There is another wise saying: 'When you're young, you've got a girl but no couch. Later on'—at my age, for instance—'you've got the couch but no girl.' Look for a new girl. You'll find the couch. Forget the Hohengraben."

Every Sunday morning we met at the Kapuzinergruft, the crypt of the Capuchins. Since the beginning of the seventeenth century, Habsburgs had been buried here, beneath an early baroque building in the heart of Vienna. A Capuchin brother sat behind an unpolished desk in the entrance hall, meditatively stroking his little beard and collecting the admission fees. He always gave me an approving glance. "You are a good young man," he observed once. "You come to visit the crypt regularly after morning mass."

There was a side entrance to the little church. "We must be careful," Liesl said. "My father's eyes are quite capable of seeing me from Graz"—a hundred and fifty kilometers away. "He frowned even at the idea of my meeting a Berkovitzki, when Uncle wrote to him about you. 'I am warning you now, Liesl,' father wrote. 'Never go out without a female escort. I know those Berkovitzkis. Eighteenth-century nobility!' "

For hours we walked around the crypt, until I could have served as an extraordinarily well-informed guide, because as we talked and whispered or stood in a silent embrace, almost inevitably I would find myself reading the inscription on the nearest tomb. I came to know all those pious legends by heart, from that on the sarcophagus of Emperor Matthias and his wife—the founding couple—to Emperor Franz Josef's. Whispering, kissing, or simply looking into each other's eyes, we breathed the incense in the air and the scent of wax candles. Those scents, and the feeling of that holy and—for me—love-drenched atmosphere, would still be in the air as I pored over my books and dissected and stared into the microscope and made innumerable blood counts at the physiology lab.

She would persuade her father somehow, Liesl said. She said it again and again, at the Kapuzinergruft, at the Opern Café, and in the tall, frosty room with the baroque windows and the piano with the faintly yellowed keys. "I'm his only child. He *can't* make me unhappy," she sobbed at our last rendezvous in the crypt. We were standing beside the casket of the Duke of Reichstadt, the son of Napoleon.

iii

THE GENERAL HOSPITAL...
AND VERA

So read the inscription over the entrance to the Allgemeines Krankenhaus. Can I ever forget the moment when I first came through those doors of the General Hospital as a full-fledged student of clinical medicine? The basic sciences were very important, of course, but now real life would begin—seeing living patients, examining them, learning how to prescribe.

Josef II, the enlightened Habsburg, had built the hospital. Since then a few buildings had been added, but in my time it looked more or less the same: small buildings separated by courtyards with patches of green. The incense here was iodine and carbolic acid; in the spring these harsh odors were softened by the scent of blossoming acacia trees.

But now it was October. Father had regained his old position as administrator of the Workers' Sick Benefit Panel of the Province of Burgenland, since the western part of Hungary had been ceded to Austria by the Treaty of St. Germain. I had spent the

long summer vacation near St. Gilgen, that magnificent town on
the western shore of the Wolfgangsee, serving as a doctor's aide in
a camp for teen-age apprentices. I served also as lifeguard; I was a
good swimmer and easily passed the qualifying examination. The
camp was a three-hour walk from St. Gilgen. Several times a week
I would set out with a dozen boys along the mountain roads that
wound through pine forests. In the crisp, delicious air the sun-
light fell in stripes across the aromatic shadows and sparkled on
the grass and wildflowers. When we were almost at St. Gilgen, the
church tower would come in sight, then the lake itself, and in
seconds we had pulled off our clothes and jumped into swimming-
suits and plunged with gasps and shouts into the icy mountain
water.

There was only one thing wrong with my summer vacation,
and it became increasingly worse: I had no news from Liesl. Before we separated at the casket of the Duke of Reichstadt—leaving by separate exits because of her father's far-seeing eyes—she
promised to write at least once a week and instructed me to write
poste restante to the main post office in Graz, not to her home. I
wrote one letter after another. The old mailman with mustache *à
la* Franz Josef who came to the camp looked pityingly at me as he
shook his head: *kein Brief.* What was wrong? Was she ill? Had
she confessed to her father? Had he threatened her, forced her to
promise to break off and not even write? Days and weeks, weeks
and weeks—and only silence. There were plenty of girls around,
nurses at the camp, girls in town, and everybody had a girl friend.
Not I. The boys began to tease me: "Is there something wrong
with you?"

But youth is indestructible, and I couldn't deny that I felt fine
when I visited my parents at the end of summer, before returning
to Vienna. They were living in Sauerbrunn, seat of the Burgenland provincial government. Mother's eyes rested with satisfaction on her tanned and well-fed son.

The very day I got back to Vienna I took the trolley out to the

Schönbrunnerstrasse. The gardens seemed even more neglected; the front door was unlocked, as always. My heart pounded as I hurried in, listening for piano music. There was nobody at the piano in her room; there was no sign of her, not even a hint of her perfume in the air. I went looking for her uncle and found him at his desk, of course, looking like a shriveled apple, working away at the memoirs. He noticed me only when I touched his shoulder. Then, glancing up over his spectacles, his eyes expressed joy. "What an honor!" he exclaimed. "The Duke of Krapfenberg! Or his son—or are you even his grandson? There is a striking family resemblance. Such a coincidence! I'm just revising the files of the Ministry in the 1890s. Here, look, you can see your father's or grandfather's handwriting. We were in the same department, you know."

"Where is Elisabeth?" I shouted. He smiled radiantly. I put my mouth next to his ear and yelled in a voice that could have been heard in Graz, "WHERE IS ELIZABETH?"

"Yes, I assure you it is a fact," he replied, beaming. "We were in the same department for years." He had become stone deaf.

I wrote my question on a piece of paper. He read it, frowned, shook his head. "I haven't heard from her since she went to Graz for the summer vacation."

I left.

I went to the Kapuzinergruft. The monk in the entrance hall smiled and nodded. "Ah, the pious young gentleman. So glad to see you. Where is your worthy sister?"

I walked through the crypt from tomb to tomb and smelled the incense and the wax candles but no trace of Elisabeth's perfume, not even by the casket of the Duke of Reichstadt.

"You look excellent," Herr Franz said, "tanned. And you have gained weight." I ordered two soft-boiled eggs and buttered rolls. He brought them and inspected me. "But why so gloomy? Is it the Hohengraben girl?"

"Yes," I said and told him the story.

"Hmm," he said, biting his mustache. "Didn't I warn you about her father, those cruel eyes? *Ja,* these high-ranking people, they know what to do with a naughty girl—send her to Paris or London or Rome, make her forget her sweetheart the commoner. D'you think *they* realize that times have changed, that we're living in a republic, that there aren't any special privileges? That His Imperial Majesty is in exile? *'Der Kaiser geht, die Generäle bleiben,'* that's what they're saying in Germany, and it also goes for us. They are here to stay, those people. I'm no Communist, as you know, but it burns me up. Is a doctor less than one of those blue-blooded nincompoops?"

Sadly I agreed. "But how can I get in touch with her, Herr Franz?"

"Forget it, *Herr Doktor.* There are millions of girls around."

Can any doctor forget when he first placed a stethoscope on a patient's chest and listened to the sounds of breathing and the sounds of the beating heart? It was some time before one could tell the normal from the pathological: vesicular, bronchial breathing; wheezing; rales; heart murmurs. Surgery: the operating room with its special aroma of chloroform and ether. Obstetrics: the newborn baby's outraged cry. Ophthalmology: conjunctivitis, trachoma, cataract; examination of the eye-ground. Gonorrhea; syphilis. Psychiatry: dementia praecox. Pharmacology: Rx. Ear, nose, and throat. Pediatrics: diphtheria, whooping cough, scarlet fever, mumps. Hygiene. Forensic medicine.

And post mortems at the Institute of Pathology.

I walked from building to building of the teaching hospital. The wall surrounding it separated the world of the healthy from the world of disease and pain. In this small walled city, this fortress, truly we were in a world of our own.

Almost a hundred and fifty years before, in 1777, Joseph II, the son of Maria Theresa, traveled from Vienna to Paris, bearing a stern letter from his mother warning her frivolous daughter Marie Antoinette to behave herself. Rumors had reached Vienna that the French were outraged by the behavior of their queen, who threw money away while people starved. Joseph added warnings and admonitions of his own. The splendors of Paris and Versailles were quite a change for him, who came from rather frugal Vienna. He was fascinated by the Hôtel Dieu and decided that, back in Vienna, he would build the most modern hospital in Europe.

He was hampered by those same "high-ranking" people Herr Franz had castigated, who were jealous and suspicious of anything stemming from Paris, but seven years later the great feat was accomplished. Writers of the time marveled at the extensive hospital departments and paid tribute to Joseph, the enlightened monarch.

It was impossible not to be impressed by the solemn, unique, and glorious history of medicine in Vienna. Learning as much as I did about it during my medical-student years, sometimes I seemed to be living in the eighteenth and early nineteenth centuries. I came to feel that only yesterday, or the day before yesterday, Johann Peter Frank, the hospital's most famous director, had walked those same halls. He established pathology as an independent discipline and treated Napoleon after the conquest of Vienna in 1809. (One of our professors said that Frank had diagnosed the illness which later killed the Emperor; how interesting it would be if Frank's notes of the examination could be found!) Frank loved music, which was a tradition among Viennese physicians (a doctor making a house call was expected by the patient to tell him the name of the opera that had been performed the day before); in his home, the *Gartenschlössl* in the Alserstrasse near the hospital, his best friend, Haydn, often visited him, and, later, Beethoven. Mozart had been treated by a competitor, Matthias Sallaba, also a professor at the teaching hospital.

Back in those years I learned procedures which seemed to be

simple; percussion and auscultation, which today young people
take for granted. Weren't they known and practiced thousands
and thousands of years ago? In the auditorium I listened to
stocky, bespectacled Franz Chvostek, one of the most eloquent
and fiery teachers of internal medicine. He spoke of percussion
and auscultation as fairly recent discoveries. Leopold Auenbrugger von Auenbrugg described the procedures in 1761. He was the
son of an innkeeper and he noticed that empty wine barrels and
full barrels make quite different sounds when tapped with the
fingers. A barrel somewhat resembles a human chest; Leopold
Auenbrugger began to tap chests. Normal lung tissue, filled with
air, makes one kind of sound; the airless tissue of pathology
makes quite another.

But Auenbrugger's discovery was ignored and forgotten—"a
typical Austrian destiny," Chvostek observed. "One of his con-
temporaries said, 'Who has ever heard of pneumonia playing music?' and everyone laughed. But forty years later, when the French-
men Lennaec and Corvisart rediscovered the secret of the wine
barrels—well! Then suddenly our good Viennese friends believed
it." And Chvostek snapped his fingers to demonstrate contempt
for "our good Viennese friends" and rolled down his cuffs.

His shirt cuffs often rolled up and down his arms as he listened
to the patient's chest and gestured and thundered his observations to us. From him I first heard the word "hyperthyroidism."
The son of a world-famous physician (the "Chvostek sign" in tetanus was named for his father), he lived up to his father's reputation as a clinician. When he lectured and demonstrated, the auditorium was always crammed. He was implacably against women
in medicine. *"In der Küchen, in der Kirchen, mit Kinder, ja"*—
but not as physicians. Otherwise he was understanding and won-
derfully tolerant of his students' ignorance. "I don't know much
more than you do," he would shout. It counted practically as a
miracle to flunk one of his exams (I achieved the miracle).

Karl Friedrich Wenckebach, the most famous cardiologist of

the day, was an entirely different personality, erect, always elegantly dressed, soft-spoken. In his auditorium we saw a giant machine (a giant, that is to say, in comparison with the machines to which it would lead), the original electrocardiograph. An electrode was placed on each of the subject's forearms, and one on the left leg; with a mysterious whirring and ticking the machine began to operate, and zigzag lines on small stripes wrote the electrocardiogram. "By this method one can detect arryhthmias," Wenckebach explained. (In his book, published in 1921, he stated this. Later he was one of the cardiologists whose attention was drawn to peculiarities shown on those lines; deviations, up-and-downward deflections: the "P" waves, the "T" waves, the "Q" waves, the diagnostic criteria of myocardial damage, heart attacks. I did not learn about the present twelve-lead EKG until twenty years later, in America.)

"Forget it," was Herr Franz's advice, but how could I forget Liesl—her cameo face, almost transparently pale, the thin child-like fingers, trembling slightly when she caressed me, and the music and the shadowy old room with baroque windows? Until I met her, music had been simply a distraction, a romantic, somewhat sentimental amusement; she taught me to understand it. As we stood in the scented half-darkness of the Kapuzinergruft she told me about the history of music. I can hear her whispering voice: secular music, the troubadours and *Minnesängers* of the early Middle Ages; the organists at Notre Dame, and the thirteenth-century English musician Walter de Odington. I recall the sunsets as we looked out from her room in the Schönbrunner-strasse and she described the Dutch school and Guillaume Dufay, and the baroque (my eternal love for the baroque was given to me by Liesl), and Palestrina, and Orlando di Lasso, and counterpoint. She told me about the great violin-makers, Nicolò Amato and Stradivari. And: "Did you know this, Richard? Opera is really a quite recent musical gentre—seventeenth century. The

earliest opera, *Euridice,* was composed by the Florentine Peri.
She explained the difference between an aria and a recitative. I
had never quite been able to tell the difference between Handel's
music and Bach's; she made it clear. She talked about Monteverdi,
Stradella, Scarlatti, Henry Purcell, and Milton, and went to the
piano and played a few notes of their music. She agreed with
Rossini that Beethoven was the *greatest* musician in history—"but
nevertheless," she added, smiling, "Mozart was the *only* one." Her
deer-brown eyes seemed to glow over the yellowed keys as she
played a little Mozart. She admired Richard Strauss. "The Viennese didn't appreciate his *Salomé,*" she said. "The Viennese are
always deprecating. To deprecate is a Viennese talent."

It is all very well to live in memories and weep at the sound of
certain music, and feel the heart pound when a girl's ash-blond
head appears in the crowds standing at the opera (never hers),
but it is not enough.

On a December night in 1924 Bruno Walter conducted Mozart's *Requiem* in memory of Giacomo Puccini, who had died
that day. (Thirty-three years later my son and I went to hear *La
Bohème* at the Metropolitan Opera House in New York. The
performance stopped; Rudolf Bing came out and announced that
Arturo Toscanini was dead. The lights went down, and Dimitri
Mitropoulos conducted the prelude to the third act of *La Travi-
ata.*) Puccini had been a familiar figure in Vienna and was deeply
loved. You could hear the sound of sobs in the Konzerthaussaal.
Indeed someone was crying right next to me. It was a girl. She
leaned on my shoulder a little bit, and we walked out together,
but I was thinking of Liesl.

Then I saw the same girl at the opera, and again at a concert.
She was really quite beautiful, with a healthy complexion—about
eighteen, I thought; maroon hair and pigtails. I saw her again at
the opera, and we introduced ourselves. Her name was Vera. She
spoke in a good strong voice and made large gestures. She was a
dramatic student at the Reinhardt Seminar, where of course they

paid attention to the voice and to appropriate gestures. We went to the Josefstädtertheater, where modern plays were performed—Molnár, Henry Bernstein. "At school," Vera said, "we are rehearsing *Liliom*."

I remember that night very well because for the first time she took me to her apartment, in the Berggasse, not far from where Freud lived. We climbed up three flights on tiptoe and crept into the apartment. Vera struck a match and put it to a candle. "It is not advisable to make any noise coming up the stairs, because the landlady has the ears of an elephant," she told me. "Also it isn't advisable to have any more light; the old devil can trace it through the door cracks, even though she's two rooms away."

Her large blue eyes blinked at me when I put my arms around her and kissed her. She said she had invited me here to rehearse, but she understood. Later she produced a large woven basket filled with giant apples her parents had sent her. They lived in Salzburg; her father was a teacher. We ate apples with gusto and spoke about the future: I wanted to become a surgeon, Vera hoped to act at the Burgtheater.

I studied obstetrics, and she rehearsed *Liliom*.

I told her with pride (all our conversations were in a low key because of the landlady's hearing powers) about the delivery room. "You put the stethoscope on the mother's abdomen and listen to the baby's rapid heart sounds. This is the sequence of events: a small vortex appears at the vulva, followed by the whole skull, and then the wrinkled little face, and the baby's first yell."

What I didn't tell her were the difficulties I had encountered during my first steps in obstetrics. Before we were permitted to examine a genuine pregnant woman nearing term, we had to practice on a dummy, which we called "the phantom." Everything was simple. We put our fingers into the imitation vagina and ascertained the imitation baby's position. Through the imitation abdominal wall we felt the body parts and learned from imitation abnormal positions the technique of rotating the baby so that normal delivery could be achieved. Once there was an imitation pelvic presentation, and I got myself ready to perform the prescribed maneuver when, to my horror, I saw the gentlemanly face of Professor Kermauner watching me. With trembling fingers I turned the imitation baby in all directions, but I could not extricate it. Kermauner took over; in a few seconds all was well, imitation delivery accomplished. He smiled at me. "Be careful," he said, "or next time the mother will change to another obstetrician."

In the actual delivery room, everything was difficult. Gowned and masked, we felt as if we were in a steambath. A genuine abdomen is not so easy to handle as the rubber belly of a dummy, and it took time to be able to recognize a real baby's heart sounds and to differentiate the smooth round head from the smooth round buttocks.

Herr Franz was pleased with my new choice. When Vera first entered the Café Klinik, all eyes turned to her—not just students', but old eyes, professors' eyes, peering up from their papers and lingering on the fine firm young body.

During my period of grief, of tears at the sound of music once heard in a shadowy old room, Herr Franz had tried to be helpful. At eleven at night in the Café Klinik the scenery changed, so to speak; the students departed, and the night clientele came in, the whores from the Gürtel—very tired, heads dropping down to rest on their breasts. Herr Franz was on good terms with them, and one after another they would come to my table. *"Bubi,* even a big scholar like you should have a bit of fun, *nicht wahr?"*

Now again I had a girl friend. Was it love? Vera was a warm, full-fledged, cooperative, thoughtful female. And she was much prettier than Liesl and did not believe in waiting until after marriage. Still, something was missing. My friends envied me and seemed to feel that somehow things weren't right, I didn't deserve this beautiful girl. Why not? What was so exceptional about the situation? I can still see myself, tall, thin, with disheveled brown hair (and a few streaks of gray, which had first appeared when I was eighteen). Herr Franz explained it. *"Die Weiber san halt blöd,"* he said, smiling with satisfaction. "Women are stupid."

Bit by bit I had ingratiated myself with Vera's landlady, Frau Koglbauer, the human elephant, and she now accepted me, with certain reservations. "He's a nice young fellow," I heard her saying to Vera. *"Schade* that he's Jewish."

By this time we were meeting every night. During the days Vera was at her dramatic school and I in the hospital departments. I never missed the surgical lectures; it is only the very rare medical student whose first love is not surgery. Billroth, the greatest surgeon of the age, had died twenty-five years before; our professor, Hochenegg, quoted him on every occasion. "Surgery is the one discipline in medicine which you can really grasp," Billroth had said. Before his time, abdominal surgery had been taboo; appendicitis was treated by medication, almost invariably with fatal results.

We watched Professor Hochenegg operate in the amphitheater. He was a brilliant lecturer. He still relied first on the clinical impression, before using X rays. The Kraske-Hochenegg operation, removal of a rectum carcinoma, is the accepted method to this day.

Tall, heavy-set, with a substantial paunch, gesticulating, stroking his long beard, he liked to tell anecdotes drawn from his and his colleagues' practice. "A lady approached my friend and asked him if the appendix was an essential organ. 'Definitely, madam,' he replied, 'for the surgeon.' " He had a whole catalogue of jokes about clerical patients. "There was this priest from a little town out in the woods somewhere who came to me for the removal of his diseased gall bladder. 'Once more our good Lord has helped His humble servant,' he said piously just before he left, and folded his hands and raised his eyes to heaven. 'Well,' I said, 'I'm damned if I know why He couldn't have helped you while you were still at home, instead of making you come all this way.' "

But often enough Hochenegg was in no mood for jokes. Can one visualize an operation today without blood ready for transfusion? Sometimes the patient became paler and paler while the operation was in progress. "The operation was a success, but the patient died." Old Hochenegg's giant head would drop; he would lift his hands in a gesture of helplessness.

Thirty years later, when my son was studying medicine in Chicago, I admired the diligence of those young men who for four irretrievable years buried themselves in books, in laboratories— four years of youth gone forever! How different it had been with us. After finishing the basic sciences, we had two and a half years of relative freedom, when no one forced us to attend lectures; "academic freedom" *was* freedom. I would not have traded those years for anything—golden years, when Vienna was Vienna, a big city embedded among gardens, surrounded by castled hills with vineyards on the slopes. And there were cafés at every corner, where we sat and watched the girls in the springtime, when Vienna was one giant flower garden.

Vera and I didn't have much money; her father, a teacher, and mine, a civil servant, were in no position to support us lavishly. But she had connections with some of the theaters, and occasionally they needed extras. We appeared in operas, straight plays, comedies, and farces, in a multitude of costumes and a colorful variety of make-up—tiny bit parts, paying tiny salaries. We didn't have a car; we had our strong young legs. We wandered up the hills and in winter skated on the frozen Danube. For a few groschen we could spend the night in a *Schutzhütte* on a mountaintop two or three thousand meters high. I can see Vera's flushed face and half-frozen nose and hear her broad laughter. We were breathing hard when we reached the top of the Schneeberg, the Rax, and looked far down into the valley. We made love in the thin, biting air and ate with good appetite our Butterbrot, tasty corn-and-rye bread, and chewed on a huge hunk of salami.

Finally Frau Koglbauer became resigned to the fact that I spent whole nights with her young lady roomer. *"Ja, das ist die Jugend,"* she would murmur when she saw me bounding down the stairs at eight in the morning. "He runs like a deer." For Christmas, 1924, I bought her a tiny Madonna and Child. She, of the elephant ears and X-ray sight, was a tiny old lady who wore a brown kerchief; and I remember that after she took the Madonna and put it down and admired it she tightened the kerchief and showed me her toothless mouth in a broad smile. "There are nice Jews," she said.

When Herr Franz brought me a cup of coffee and a piece of Gugelhupf one morning, I saw that his face looked worn and lined. It was useless, I knew, to ask him if anything was wrong; he had often told me that the Allgemeines Krankenhaus hadn't been built for him and that *he* would never seek shelter in the hospital's morgue (a pleasant view that could be seen from the Café Klinik).

But late that night, around midnight, when even the whores were beginning to thin out, he came to my table and spoke solemnly. *"Herr Doktor,* are you ready to—look me over?"

Here was a tremendous compliment for a last-year medical student—the first "private patient!" He beckoned, and I followed him through the kitchen, which I had never entered before, to a little room with shelves laden with eggs and butter, hams, sausages, bread, cakes. There was also a small bench. "Lie down, please, Herr Franz," I said.

He lay down. "It hurts me here," he said, "like cramps." And he pointed to his abdomen.

I made the diagnosis. "Gall-bladder disease," I told him. "You need a work-up, X rays and so on."

"Oh, *nein!* Nature will take care." He narrowed his beagle eyes.

"Nature will not take care, Herr Franz. You must get it over with."

"Only once before, in all my life," he said, "was I examined by a doctor, and even then it wasn't genuine. I mean I was malingering—a *Tachenierer,* they called it in the Army. I imitated a terrible chest cold, and the *Regimentsarzt,* a good-natured captain, sent me to the hospital. I bribed an orderly and spent the nights with my lady friend, who was an excellent cook."

"This time you're not malingering, Herr Franz, and you are going to have the work-up."

He sighed. "Oh well, you could be right. And I would not offend a young doctor."

His gall bladder was filled with stones. I was permitted to watch the operation, a singular honor for a medical student. Three weeks later he was discharged from the hospital. The wound wasn't completely healed, and Professor Hochenegg, who had confirmed my diagnosis, told me to look after it. "I knew Franz when we were both young," he said with a melancholy smile. "Clean the wound every day, don't forget the Peru balsam" —antibiotics and chemotherapy were a quarter of a century in the future—"then put on a good dressing."

Herr Franz lived in a little room on the top floor of an ancient house in the Pramergasse. His beagle eyes anxiously followed my every move as I cleaned and dressed the wound. *"Sehr gut,"* he commented. "Much gentler than those damned nurses. But perhaps they're good in the bed."

On the otherwise bare walls there were half a dozen striking color lithographs of elegant ladies in huge ostrich hats, *fin-de-siècle* pin-up girls. He saw me looking at them. "Two divorces," he confessed. "I always had enough. There is a song, *Herr Doktor:* 'When you're young the world is yours. Later it costs money.' "

iv

THE PROFESSORS

Two great specialists, Heinrich Neumann and Maximilian Hayek, lectured on diseases of the ear, nose, and throat. Their specialization was even narrower: Neumann specialized in the ear and nose, Hayek in the throat. They were Hungarian Jews who had risen to worldwide fame in Vienna; Neumann had been knighted, and in higher Jewish circles his name and honor were used as an irrefutable argument in favor of the proposition that anti-Semitism was a thing of the past. (Later, a refugee, he died and was buried in New York.)

They profoundly disliked each other and would not teach in the same building, so two separate hospitals were established. Hayek's was additionally famous among us students. Fuel was scarce in postwar Vienna; sometimes even the Café Klinik was so cold you could see your breath, and of course the rooming houses were freezing; but in the cellar of Hayek's hospital the blessed steam-heat pipes crisscrossed the ceiling and breathed a gentle tropical heat on the hundreds of students crammed below. The "Hayek *Keller*" became as famous as the Herr Professor. Many a night I fell asleep there over my books.

ENT was a predominantly surgical domain in my day, because of course there were no antibiotics for treating infections. An inflamed eardrum signaled a serious disease and had to be punctured in time, because if the accumulated pus wasn't released the inner ear would become infected, and often the mastoid bone. Or the infection might reach the brain, frequently with a fatal result. One can still see people with the telltale scar above the mastoid bone, souvenir of a long-ago ear operation.

Neumann was a squarely built man in his late fifties. An excellent teacher with an exuberant temperament, he always lectured to a full auditorium. The imposing reflector flashed on his forehead as he strode around and gestured and, in the voice of a Shakespearean actor, described the slings and arrows of outrageous fortune that might strike the nose and ear; but then suddenly his Austrian-German accent would change into Hungarian-Yiddish, and his fleshy lips would curl up and writhe in pure pleasure as he pronounced the punch line of a favorite joke. We were always waiting for those jokes; sometimes the lecture hour consisted of little else, and the auditorium rang with laughter.

Neumann's hero was a famous Hungarian surgeon of his student days, Professor Baron of Budapest. Here is a story.

"A stingy millionaire bargained with Baron about the operation fee. Finally the professor lost his patience. 'If my fee is too high for you, why don't you let one of my assistants do the job? They're good too.' 'But Herr Professor,' said the millionaire, 'you are renowned for your steady hands.' 'And how can they be steady if they're trembling for the fee?' Baron asked."

Another: "Two Hungarian businessmen met in a Viennese café to discuss trade secrets. Of course they spoke in Hungarian. In comes a typical Viennese business type, ruddy, smoking a big cigar, sits down at the next table, and begins to read the paper. The two Hungarians frowned suspiciously at each other: was the newcomer a spy? Could he understand Hungarian? How to find out? Ask him? Ridiculous. How? The smarter Hungarian got a bright idea. He leaned over to the neighboring table, tapped the Viennese gentleman's paper. 'Excuse me,' he whispered in Hungarian, 'but your fly is wide open.' The cunning gentleman's hand flew to his trousers. 'Thank you,' he muttered."

Maximilian Hayek was a little man with a neat, tiny beard. He was one of the founders of modern speech therapy; his rehabilitation program after surgical removal of the larynx is still used (one of his former assistants practices it in New York today). His lectures were not easy to follow; he had none of Neumann's eloquence or sense of humor, and his knowledge of nonmedical literature was negligible. The Vienna of my day was abundantly supplied with famous writers, but when Arthur Schnitzler the novelist telephoned Hayek and introduced himself and then said that his colleague Franz Kafka had a serious condition of the larynx and was in need of immediate hospitalization, Hayek looked puzzled. "He seemed to think I should know who he was," he remarked later. "Schnitzler? Who is Schnitzler? Who is this Kafka?"

The Vienna of my day was also abundantly supplied with anti-Semitism; so-called "modern," racial anti-Semitism originated there. It emerged twice a year, virulently, at the university at registration time. Nationalist and clerical students tried to stop Jews from coming in—a kind of carnival watched by hundreds of Viennese. It was wiser to wait, if you were a Jew, until the *Studentenkravalle* abated. I had been in one brawl, and when I tried to register for the last semester I got into another. An unpleasant fellow wearing the cap of the nationalist student society stopped me. "Let's see your credentials," he said.

I have a Semitic face—at any rate, a prominent nose—but I wasn't usually taken for a Jew, probably because of my provincial accent when speaking German. "None of your business," I said.

"We're just checking on Jews," he explained with a fraternal smile.

"I am a Jew," I said. "Get out of my way."

"What!" he said. "Why, you damn kike!"

I was muscular from much swimming, soccer-playing, and other athletic activities, and I started to punch him in his Christian nose, but unfortunately one corner of my heavy gynecology atlas somehow became involved and hit him below the left eye. Blood spurted out of a gaping wound. The sight of blood was too much for him, and he fainted. A gang of his friends surrounded me, and I would have been beaten up if proctors' men hadn't interfered.

The dean suspended me and threatened to report me to the police. My final destiny was to be decided by the *Professorenkollegium*.

"What you did was right!" Herr Franz said. "That *Schweinehund* will think a couple of times in the future before he tries to stop someone."

"I'm in a lot of trouble," I said, "and just before starting my finals."

"*Mir wearn scha sehn,*" Herr Franz said with a promising gesture.

"You should have killed the bastard," Vera said later.

I was sitting on her bed, somberly eating an apple. "You have just had another demonstration of what upper-class Jewish circles are always telling one another," I said. " 'Jews are equal citizens.' "

"Of course they are. Just because a few lice act like gangsters—"

"Would you marry me?"

"Naturally I would!"

"What would your father say—a Catholic parochial schoolteacher?"

"He tried to stop me from becoming an actress and he didn't, did he?"

"Marriage is something else."

"I wouldn't give a damn what he said!"

I finished the apple. "Please cheer up," she said.

When I left, Frau Koglbauer saw my gloomy face. "You must not be so sad, *Herr Doktor*," she said. "There is always a silver lining."

It was April, a beautiful sunny day. I sat on a bench in the Votivpark, facing on one hand the twin towers of the Votivkirche, on the other a university building. I watched the students streaming out. My lousy rotten temper, I thought; why couldn't I have kept away from the university on registration day and registered later? Could I alone change the goddamn world? Was it my business to eliminate somehow the anti-Semitism little children sucked in with their mothers' milk? Here I was, sitting on a park bench, just before the end of years of study—now all for nothing, all sacrifices in vain. The young lout whose cheek my gynecology atlas had opened up had fully recovered, but I would never be forgiven.

For the past few days Herr Franz had been missing at intervals from the Café Klinik, but the night of that April day—a day of utter despair—he was present. With two boiled eggs and a buttered roll he also served me a small note. It was from the dean's office; it read: "The *Professorenkollegium* has decided that the case of R.B. will be dropped—for the time being. If it should ever happen again . . ."

Herr Franz was nibbling at his mustache. "Sometimes," he said, "we little people also have our channels."

Clemens von Pirquet was our chief of pediatrics. A rather slight man in his late forties, the descendant of French aristocrats who had fled the Revolution, he had a truly cosmopolitan spirit. He was a native Viennese; after graduation he had left for Johns Hopkins University in Baltimore, where he did research in skin reactions and discovered a reaction to which he gave the name "allergy." From that time on his reputation spread. He was called back to Vienna to occupy the much coveted chair of pediatrics, and he accepted the invitation, but his heart, it seemed, stayed at Johns Hopkins. The famous Dr. William H. Welch, his friend and mentor, wanted him to return and tried to persuade the Board of Regents to give Pirquet the salary of $10,000 he had asked for (while proposing to give any income from private patients to the medical school); the Board of Regents said no. Pirquet remained in Vienna.

In his immaculate lecture room we listened to Pirquet explain the NEM theory by which he endeavored to establish a standard of food, or nourishment, values—long since replaced by the much simpler method of calories. He showed us innumerable cases of measles, whooping cough, scarlet fever, mumps. We saw the grayish membrane that covered the tonsils and adjoining areas of diphtheria patients; the inoculation to prevent that dread disease was developed a decade later. We listened to his quiet voice explaining the skin reaction of tuberculosis; the Pirquet test is still used, in modified form, to detect tubercular infections even when there are no clinical or radiological signs of the disease. Another of his merits, no less valuable, lay in quite another sphere: after the war, when famine threatened tens of thousands of babies in Vienna, Pirquet used his special American connections and procured tons of milk.

Pediatrics became an important part of my practice as a country doctor. When a panicky mother awakened me at two a.m. with the information that her baby had no appetite, the mild face of Pirquet would appear before my eyes and again I would hear his soft voice: "Treating babies is simple. Dealing with their mothers is an art. You must learn to be an artist—of patience."

At fifty-five, this gentle person committed suicide. I have often wondered: was it nostalgia for Baltimore or the memory of his defeat by the Board of Regents?

As often as our meager budget permitted, Vera and I went to the opera and the other theaters; for her, this was part of her curriculum. We stood close together in the packed standing room; her maroon locks tickled my cheek; my hands touched her strong, full bosom; I deeply inhaled her sweet breath. Then in her room we would discuss the evening's performances: *die* Jeritza, Piccaver, Richard Mayr—certainly he was the best Ochs von Lerchenau in *Der Rosenkavalier*. At Max Reinhardt's experimental theater we saw Schnitzler's *Anatol*, a shocking event for conservative Viennese circles. I studied psychiatry, pathology, ophthalmology, while Vera walked up and down reciting Shakespeare, Molnár, Shaw. I thought she was very talented.

We wanted to get married, the sooner the better. Before long she would graduate and go to work as a professional actress. I still had a year of medical school ahead, to be followed by hospital training, but with what she would earn and contributions from my family, we could manage. After I established a practice she would abandon her career.

I told Mother about our plans; Father left the "internal policy" of the household completely in her hands, busy as he was with his Sick Benefit Panel and as a prominent official of the Social Democratic party. I could see that the thought of my marrying a gentile girl somehow disturbed her, but she said nothing. Vera came for a visit, and Mother succumbed to her charm. One objection remained: "The husband should support the family." We should wait.

Another thought occurred to Mother. "And what about your family, my dear?" she asked Vera, who smiled. "Of course they'd never let me marry a Jew," she said. "But I'll be twenty-one soon and they won't be able to do anything about it."

The summer of 1925 was a happy time in our lives. I had a job in a children's camp near Salzburg. Vera visited me practically every weekend; we went to the festivals, saw a superb performance of *Jedermann* in the courtyard of a medieval cloister, climbed the Untersberg, the mountain where King Frederick Barbarossa lies buried, waiting to emerge in full war equipment to review his troops. Often we wandered across the slopes of the Alps and once climbed over the Almbachklam to Berchtesgaden, where a Nazi meeting was taking place. Hitler was there, a pasty-faced man in a trenchcoat, hair slicked down on one side.

On a rainy day in September we resumed our studies. I remember the rain because a surprise was waiting for Vera; although still in school, she had the offer of a small paying part at Reinhardt's theater. Of course I remember her debut. She was charming—not a trace of stage fright. There was much applause after her exit. At the party afterward Reinhardt himself said to her, "You were good," and he was notoriously stingy with compliments. It made me a bit jealous to see her courted by so many handsome men. She smiled at me, took my hand, pressed it.

The forensic-medicine lectures resembled horror movies. Bald, stout Professor Haberda circled around the grisly tables: here, a suicide by hanging; there, a man stabbed to death; here, a young woman raped and killed. Haberda explained how rape could be diagnosed, although, he added with a malicious smile, he didn't believe in rape. "Can you imagine, *meine Herren,* that a thread can be pushed through the narrow slit if the slit is yelling and jumping around? Those women!"

We doubted that forensic medicine would be of much use in our practices; how often does a doctor have to deal with murder or suicide? And yet during my years as a country practitioner one of old Haberda's lectures was vividly brought back. I was called to a peasant home deep in the Rosalia Mountains. With tears in his eyes the young man told me that when he had waked up that morning his wife was not in bed. He found her in the barn, a knife stuck in her chest. I examined the body. The knife was still there, piercing through the fabric of blouse and chemise. What had Haberda said? "Suicides never stick the blade through the fabric—always into the naked body." I reported the case to the police; the young peasant went to jail for life.

Vera was cast in a new play as the ingénue. The rehearsals started in the morning and lasted until late in the afternoon, leaving her exhausted. The opening night turned her into a star; there were pictures in the newspapers and magazines, reporters always after her, autograph-hunters. I was studying for my finals, and sometimes we didn't meet for days. Once in the morning before going to school I dropped in to her room and slipped under the blankets. She woke up and turned to me with a smile, and we made love, but toward the end she fell asleep.

On New Year's Eve I skipped an evening post mortem and waited for her to leave the theater. She was one of the last to come out. The autograph hounds besieged her, and her companion stood back with a smile. He was the leading man in the play, in his early forties, gray at the temples, with a matinee-idol mustache. Presently he took her arm and they walked to a red Daimler sports car. Vera didn't see me.

I walked toward my dormitory and on the way passed Vera's house. The Daimler was outside. I looked up and saw the tiny gleam of a candle. I could imagine their whispering voices. "We must be quiet. My landlady has the ears of an elephant."

I turned and walked back through the narrow baroque streets of the inner city and then decided to go to the Café Klinik. There was only one light, a single unshaded bulb, just as when I'd come there first, more than five years ago. There were no customers, just the shadow of one man sitting at a table. It was Herr Franz. There were three champagne bottles in front of him. I had never seen him drinking before. He looked up as the door closed behind me. "Let us celebrate together," he said in a slightly drunken voice and poured me a glass. "Drink," he said.

I drank. He put on his pince-nez and peered at me. "What is wrong?" he asked.

I told him my story.

He took off his pince-nez and shook his head. *"Ach,* these lousy women. Trash. Who the hell does she think she is? An actress— today in heaven, tomorrow nobody remembers her name! But you, you"—he waggled his finger at me—"you are a doctor! A DOCTOR! Do you understand that?" He got up decisively and walked with a military stride into the same little room where I had examined him and came back with two more bottles. He sat down firmly, almost fell, and settled himself in the chair. "Before I am too drunk, let me tell you *my* story," he said. "I have been married twice. Twice. My first wife was a waitress, tall, young, blond. A bosom like—that. One night I came home early—wait- ers do sometimes when business is slow—and found her in bed with a waiter friend. After the divorce I said to myself, 'Never marry again.' A few years later I broke my promise. This time the woman was older—a good figure, but plain. Now I thought I was safe. *Ja, ja.* One night I came home and found her in bed with a good-looking youngster from the neighborhood. You should have seen them when I came through the door! Such big eyes! My wife knew I always carried a gun at night, and she was waiting for me to pull it out. But I didn't. I just laughed, and their eyes got even bigger. I was remembering a discussion between two waiter friends: marry a pretty woman or an ugly one? 'A pretty woman, naturally,' said the first. 'Ugly,' said the second. 'Why?' asked the first. 'Because a pretty woman gets ugly; the ugly one stays the same.' "

Herr Franz drank. "I kicked her in the ass and threw the youngster out the door and watched him scampering down the street. And you?" he said. "Forget the stupid little bitch."

Although I was in the middle of my finals, I couldn't study. I had to go away for a time.

In Sauerbrunn my parents lived in a modern building with a fine garden and apple, cherry, pear, apricot, walnut trees, all bare now of course; the ground was deep in snow. For hours I wandered around the house, occasionally pausing to consume a favorite dish prepared by Mother: plum dumplings, apple strudel, and Mohnstrudel. She asked no questions. At night I went to a café where gypsies played the haunting, sad Hungarian love songs:

Csak egy kislány van a világon—
I know only one girl in the world—

Oh God, oh God. "Only one girl in the world . . ." Why had she done it? But *had* she done it? Perhaps I was mistaken. Perhaps it was someone else's Daimler. His red Daimler couldn't be the only red Daimler in Vienna. It was quite likely that somebody else had just happened to park *his* red Daimler outside Vera's house. I would go and ask her, and she would tell me that of course that was right, and we would make love.

No, I wouldn't. She had betrayed me. Night after night I listened to the sad music and got drunk.

After two weeks I had had enough gypsy music and hangovers and decided to return to Vienna and my finals. Mother went with me to the station. She hadn't been well; her diabetes was taking its toll. Her brown eyes looked at me from her thin face, and she put her hand on my cheek.

"Success isn't a good adviser; only setbacks make a man!" she said as the train pulled into the station.

THE PSYCHIATRIC WARD

The first psychiatric patient I interviewed was a classic case, a man of about thirty, neatly dressed, collected, calm. His answers to my questions were precisely to the point. He worked in an office, was single, had a girl friend, lived at home with his parents, got on well with them, although to be sure once in a while he disagreed with his father.

"Do you know where you are?" I asked.

"Certainly. In a psychiatric ward."

"Why are you here?"

He smiled. "A stupid story. On my way home yesterday I noticed that two men were following me. One pointed at me and said to the other, 'He stinks.' I turned back and asked him pointblank, 'Why did you say that?' He did not meet my eyes but glanced at his companion and muttered under his breath, 'Cuckoo.' I lost my temper and slapped him. A policeman arrived and pushed me around. I resisted. Another policeman came running up. They brought me to the precinct station and then here. That's all."

The ward doctor intervened. "Herr Hinteregger, you haven't eaten a thing since you've been here. Aren't you hungry?"

"Starving," Herr Hinteregger replied with a smile. "But the food's poisoned. You know that, don't you?"

Two attendants led him away. "You see how I'm treated," he observed over his shoulder.

"A typical case of *dementia praecox paranoides*," the instructor explained later. "An early stage of schizophrenia. At the beginning, deviations from normal behavior are hardly noticeable, and friends and relatives regard them merely as rather amusing little quirks of personality. Occasionally he won't eat; if asked why, he says his appetite is poor. He starts to withdraw into himself, explains that he likes to stay alone, read, listen to music. He feigns normality. Then one day he does something that can't be overlooked. And you have just seen and heard it."

The tall building with barred windows was a bleak place. Once a week I attended student rounds with the professor and saw patients who screamed, who struggled, or who sat slumped over, buried in nothingness, or stared at you with fiercely hostile eyes. What a blessing the sedatives and tranquilizers of today would have been!

Professor Wagner-Jauregg was known far beyond the borders of small postwar Austria, a Nobel Prize-winner for his malaria treatment of progressive paresis, a late stage of neurosyphilis. He was a familiar and striking sight in Vienna: tall, trim, with wide-brimmed black hat and mighty mustache, deep-seated gray eyes under bushy brows. The searching eyes and his formidable basso were the only means he possessed to calm an agitated patient.

The student rounds were attended not only by students but also by doctors and nurses. The professor asked the head nurse for a percussion hammer, used to test the reflexes. I happened to be at the end of the line, and a young nurse, rushing to bring the hammer, tripped over my foot as she squeezed past. I caught her. "Why don't you watch where you're going?" she whispered angrily. She hurried on, gave the hammer to the head nurse, who gave it to the professor.

"At least you could have said thank you," I whispered to the young nurse as she came back.

Her nurse's sea-gull hat jerked. "You have two left feet," she whispered.

I recognized her the next time: dark eyes, a rather pale face, no make-up. Either she didn't notice me or didn't want to.

After the first February rounds we bumped into each other at the exit. "Oh yes," she said. *"Doktor Perkussionshammer."*

"Hello," I said.

She wasn't wearing her sea-gull hat. She had jet-black hair, and her eyes weren't dark, as I'd thought at first; they were blue-greenish. She was tall and straight in the navy-blue nurse's coat.

"Good-by," she said and walked along the Lazarettgasse, where the psychiatric hospital stood. But she walked a little slowly. I took a chance and caught up with her.

"Where are you going?" I asked.

"Shopping and then home."

"Do you live with your people?"

"No, a girl-friend nurse."

"Couldn't you spare an hour with me? Dinner?"

"My girl friend's waiting."

"Too bad for me," I said. "I won't know what to do tonight."

"Why not study?"

"Thank you. One must always be thankful for good advice."

She smiled. "Now you're angry. A nurse must always obey a doctor's orders, mustn't she?"

"I'm only a student, but my eyesight is as good as any doctor's. You are very good-looking."

"Schmeichler. Young, very young—already he knows how to speak to women."

"You're the first nurse I've ever tried to date. Word of honor."

A brief interval.

We arrived at a house not far from the hospital. "This is where I live," she said. "I've thought about it: Should I? Shouldn't I? Will you wait ten or fifteen minutes? I'll change and tidy up."

I did not have a single penny in my pocket, so I thanked God for those ten or fifteen minutes. I galloped to the Café Klinik, a few blocks away. "Could you lend me fifty schillings, Herr Franz?" I panted.

"*Fifty* schillings? Who're you taking out, *die* Jeritza?"

"Not exactly. Please, Herr Franz."

He counted the bills in his wallet: thirty schillings. He walked to a table where I saw Dr. Wallner, an associate professor, buried in newspapers. Herr Franz bent over and whispered in his ear. Dr. Wallner nodded, looked at me—with understanding, I thought—and put his hand in his pocket.

Fifty schillings landed in my hand. "Be careful—*dö Weiber*," Herr Franz warned.

Back at her house, my nurse was looking in all directions. "I thought you'd changed your mind already," she said.

"Oh no, Fräulein—"

"Call me Anny."

She was stunning in a gray sports coat, even taller in high heels. The bright lipstick contrasted very attractively with the pale face and black hair. "What about Die drei Husaren?" I suggested—a rather swanky place.

"No, no," she said. "Let's eat at the Goldener Adler."

I protested; this was a modest *Bierstube* on the Singerstrasse. "A medical student and a nurse shouldn't be extravagant," she said. It was dark, and snow flurries were in the air; I looked around for a cab. "No," she said, "we will walk. I like to walk after work."

At the Goldener Adler the warm air was filled with goulash-and-beer smells. We got a table near a window. She ordered goulash; I did the same. "You're the first medical student I've ever dated," she said, mimicking me. "Word of honor."

"Is there anything extraordinary in that?"

"There is. I'm twenty-four and I think you must be the same."

"You look younger," I said. "But what's the difference?"

"Women should be with older men."

"Ridiculous," I said. "How is it you're not married, such a pretty girl?"

"No eligible men."

"No boy friend?"

"I'm just over the last. *Fini.*"

"So I am just in time," I said.

She looked at me. "Now listen, no misunderstandings. I'm not hungry for new adventures. Friendship only. The last was quite a traumatic affair."

"Mine was too."

"Then let's be friends. *Prosit.*" And she lifted her *Bierkrügl.* A picture of the Empress Elisabeth, who had been murdered at Lake Geneva, looked down benevolently at us.

"You believe in friendship only between the sexes?" I asked.

"I do," she said. "I'm no virgin, and certainly you aren't. We've both been raised in the conventional belief that man and woman *must.* When I was wondering if I should spend the evening with you, it was the thought of an evening with a young, idealistic man that was decisive. Was I wrong?"

"No, no," I assured her.

She narrowed her blue-green eyes. "Good. Then we can see each other, go to movies, the theater, talk—then a handshake. Won't that be nice?"

"Very nice," I said. But I liked her. I liked her better and better.

"Then tell 'a friend' all about your traumatic affair."

I told her, ending with the sight of the red Daimler and the tiny eloquent candle flame in the window. Anny put her hand on mine and asked, "And do you feel better now?"

"I think so," I said. "I think I'll be able to dissect without slaughtering the instructor tomorrow. And I'll listen seriously to the *Herr Professor* when he talks about schizophrenia, catatonia, amentia, paranoia."

She laughed. "I'm convinced!" I touched her hand. "Let's go," she said. "It's getting late."

Little by little I became accustomed to that somber building which at first had been a chamber of horrors—worse, in a way, than the dissecting rooms, where *they* were dead; here there were the living dead. Wagner-Jauregg's deep voice told the dramatic history of his subject: the "fools' tower," where psychotics were bound in chains, providing a merry show for sightseers, who brought their children on Sunday afternoons to see the fools' tricks. On the eve of the French Revolution, a French doctor named Pinel suggested a more humane approach. Insanity, he said, was a disease. His pronouncement was received with the same sneering skepticism which was to greet new ideas in the years to come, as it always had in the past; nevertheless, under the influence of Voltaire and Rousseau's ideas, eventually the chains came off. In Vienna ("We Viennese learn slowly," Wagner-Jauregg observed) another half-century was required to get rid of them.

Today one would call Wagner-Jauregg a conservative liberal. He foresaw the time when psychosis would be treated by medication. He did not believe in the teachings of Breuer, Freud, Alfred Adler; not once in his lectures did I hear their names. This may seem strange, in Vienna of all places. All through my life in America, if a patient or friend heard that I was a graduate of the Vienna Medical School, questions about Freud and Adler almost inevitably followed. Vienna, psychoanalysis, individual psychology—weren't they synonymous? In the sense of acceptance, they were not! I did not come in touch with modern psychiatry until much later, in France and then in the United States. (I took a "training analysis" preparatory to becoming a practicing psychiatrist in the late 1950s, but I did not, finally, become one.)

I actually saw Freud at close quarters twice in my life. After the Anschluss, the secretary of the Vienna Psychoanalytical Society—an aunt of my wife—asked him to use his world-wide influence to get visas for my family and me so we could escape from Austria. He spoke to Marie Bonaparte, a noted French psychoanalyst—great-great-great-granddaughter of Jérôme Bonaparte, Napoleon's brother—and she intervened on our behalf at the French embassy in Vienna. I went to the Berggasse to thank Freud. He received me in a small room with bookshelves around the walls, and with his old man's eyes looked at me over his spectacles while I gave a short speech. *"Schön, schön,"* he said and gave me his hand.

The second time, I was in Paris, in Marie Bonaparte's house, where he spent a day before he left for London. I asked Madame Bonaparte if I might meet Freud again. She took me to a room, knocked on the door a few times, and then cautiously opened the door. The old man, sitting in an easy chair with a book in his hands, was asleep.

Freud loved Vienna—he would have said "a love-hate relationship." *"Wien kann mich zur Raserei* [frenzy] *bringen,* but I would like to be buried here," he often said. His wish was not granted. He died in London, in exile, in 1940. At his graveside Stefan Zweig spoke in German, and H. G. Wells in English.

Anny and I began to part with more than a handshake.

"I don't know what attracted me to you," she said one night in the small room she shared with her girl friend. (One of them got home late every other night.) "You aren't what I'd call handsome. I think it was your eyes, small and urgent, like a goblin's."

"It doesn't matter why," I said.

"It does. Because your eyes lied," she said warmly. "They spoke of lots of experience, but your love-making was awkward. Oh, I know you've had *experience*, but why didn't those women teach you? That little whore at the Parhammerplatz, God knows she must have known what it's all about. And Vera—she was no virgin. With the countess, of course, you didn't even try. It's my bad luck. I had to teach you."

She would put her pink nightgown over the table lamp because it gave a dim romantic light for love-making. In between we drank brandy and smoked, while I studied psychiatry and she read *The Handbook of an Operating-Room Nurse*. She said often that she would have liked to become a doctor. Her father was a plumber with seven children; she was the fifth.

It was the spring of 1926; in the courtyards of the General Hospital the carbolic smell yielded to the lovely acacias. I would sit on a bench waiting for Anny; by and by the sea-gull cap would hurry toward me and I would feel her lips. Every other Sunday, when she was off, we would get on the trolley and travel as far as it went into the outskirts. In trenchcoats, rucksacks filled with salami, bread, cake, we wandered through the Wienerwald, and once went to the Helenenthal and from there to the little cemetery where the Baroness Vetsera, the Archduke Rudolf's tragic love, was buried. Sometimes we took the train to the Wachau valley of the Danube and climbed the hills and looked down on the river and beyond it to vineyards as far as the eye could see, with the Alps beyond.

"I'll be through with med school soon," I said. "An intern's salary isn't much, but with what you earn we could manage."

"Can't we manage now?" she said.

"I mean marriage."

"Listen," she said, "no misunderstandings! I hope you know I love you. But being sweethearts and being married are two entirely different things. Being sweethearts is a holiday. Marriage is an institution, like the government. It provides security, and you pay taxes."

I could see how satisfied she was with her explanation. "I have heard all that before," I said.

"Oh. From one of the other ladies?"

"From Herr Franz of the Café Klinik. As for the taxes, I'll pay them."

"Let's talk about something else. Look at that boat. Next time why don't we take a boat trip?"

"Let's talk about it," I said. "What's bad about me and you? Doctor and nurse—ideal combination, isn't it?"

"Later, maybe. Let me think about it. We're having such a good time, why not enjoy ourselves? Maybe tomorrow the world will blow up. Be a good boy, Richard, and let me kiss your big, beautiful Semitic nose."

In my time as a student, all examinations were oral. I can see myself in the huge amphitheater of the psychiatric hospitals, Professor Wagner-Jauregg in a chair to one side, chin resting on his black bow tie, eyes half closed, a Buddha. I, the candidate, faced the patient to be examined.

The patient was a man of about fifty, squat, with a brushlike mustache. I asked him routine questions for orientation. No response. His eyes moved around uneasily; perspiration pearls began to gather on forehead and flabby neck. His hands trembled. Suddenly he burst out, "Look, look! Look at them! Little crawling things! Mice, rats! Crawling up on you!"

It was a simple case.

Wagner-Jauregg's basso: "Are you ready?"

"I am, Herr Professor."

"Proceed."

"I have read the patient's chart. He was brought to the medical department with a gastro-intestinal hemorrhage. A chronic alcoholic, he has been deprived of alcohol since his admission. He shows a withdrawal syndrome."

"What is your diagnosis?"

"Delirium tremens."

"Wrong!" shouted the patient. "I have a Korsakoff!" (Korsakoff's syndrome is an inflammation of several nerves, occurring mostly in chronic alcoholics.)

So the patient was suddenly lucid! One corner of Wagner-Jauregg's mouth gave a little twitch; you could not quite say that he *smirked,* but I felt that he was smirking inside. *I* perspired.

The professor seemed to take pity on me. He turned to the patient. "Herr Kreitler, do you know the difference between delirium tremens and Korsakoff?"

"Nein, Herr Professor, but since I've been here so often, I know a bit of psychiatry. I get a kick out of confusing young doctors, *Herr Professor.* Sorry!" Herr Kreitler said apologetically to me.

Much to my amazement, I passed the examination.

I couldn't have looked well; when I ordered one soft-boiled egg, Herr Franz brought two, plus two pieces of Gugelhupt. "You have lost weight," he observed. "What will your mother say when she sees you? Tell her that even Herr Franz can't do anything." He took off his pince-nez and frowned. "Well, what's wrong?"

"Anny doesn't want to marry me."

"Verdammte Weiber!" he said.

"No. Anny is different."

He snorted. "Different. Once I had a colleague, a waiter at the Café Central, who came from the Trentino and often quoted an Italian writer, Pigritilli—or was it Pitigrilli? Anyway, whoever it was, Pigri or Piti, he said, 'The best love is the love you buy.' Cash. Those little whores at night, are they so bad?"

OPHTHALMOLOGY ...

AND ANNY

Professor Ernst Finger was a stately gentleman of about seventy—
he died at ninety-three—with a fine snow-white beard and elegant manners even when addressing the most ragged prostitute.
He was the head of the Department of Skin Diseases, Genitouri-
nary Diseases, and Syphilis. He had quite a sense of humor, and
his voice was thin and squeaky, which somehow made his remarks
all the funnier. Once a woman medical student was making her
first attempt to catheterize a male patient. With her trembling
left hand she tried to insert the catheter again and again. Watching the scene with evident delight, Finger asked if she was right-
handed or left-handed. "I—I am right-handed," she stammered.
"Then you must insert the catheter with your right hand," Finger
said. He narrowed his eyes. "Of course it is all right to hold the
penis in your right hand at home," he added in a remote voice.

In my memory the skin division of the department is connected
with the sight of tanks of water in which patients were immersed.
Itching, the exasperating symptom of so many skin diseases, was
most effectively treated by hydrotherapy. Now, in our time of

antibiotics, corticosteroids, antifungicides, the alleviation or even elimination of itching is much simpler.

Hundreds of patients were always waiting at the entrance to the venereal-disease out-patient clinics. Wars breed venereal disease, and World War I had left Vienna a rich legacy. Gonorrhea was treated with corrosive solutions poured into the urethra by syringe. The treatment lasted from one to two years; a single shot of penicillin can now cure the disease. As for syphilis, it was abundant in all its variations: primary, secondary, tertiary. Syphilis is still a serious problem, but again, penicillin or other antibiotics perform miracles. How many medical students of our day have seen a single case of gummata, large tumors growing out of bones and skin, the tertiary stage of syphilis?

"Ja, meine Herren, dies ist die Liebe!" And Finger pointed at a corkscrew-like spirochete, the *Treponema pallidum,* which causes syphilis, rotating on its long axis on a slide under the dark-field microscope. Hardly twenty years before, Schaudinn had discovered the pale little monster, proving that syphilis came from a microorganism; five years after that a German professor, Ehrlich, found that arsphenamine—the "magic bullet"—was effective in treating it. During my years of practice in Europe and Africa I gave thousands of intravenous arsenic injections, and also injections of bismuth, a treatment originated by Finger and used all over the world.

Finger never omitted pointing out that the venereal diseases are transmitted by sexual intercourse, and by sexual intercourse *only.* We used to tell and retell the story (perhaps it really started then; it has reproduced itself a thousand times since) of the famous person who came to Finger complaining of a discharge from the urethra. Microscopic examination proved it to be gonorrhea. "I cannot understand it, *Herr Professor,*" said the famous person. "Is it possible that I contracted it in one of those filthy toilets in our Ministry?" "Possible, Your Excellency," Finger agreed, "but damned awkward."

Anny was as unlike Liesl and Vera as a human being can be. Intellectually, and in artistic curiosity, Liesl and Vera were equals; it would have been unthinkable, impossible, for them to tell me, as Anny did, about the fainting heroines of the cloak-and-dagger love novels by Hedwig Courths Mahler. Her interest in music was restricted to the *Schrammelmusik* and the Lehár and Kálmán operettas. She had never gone to the opera—an opera company under the general management of Franz Schalk and Richard Strauss!—had never heard (oh, perhaps distantly) of Slezak, Piccaver, Jeritza, Lotte Lehmann, Elisabeth Schumann. I recall a performance of *Boris Goudonov* to which I took her. The great moment comes: Boris falls from his throne. Silence. A gentle sigh from Anny. She was asleep.

It was a delight to teach her. Her serious eyes looked straight into mine as I told her not to be discouraged, one had to learn how to enjoy music. I, an amateur, brought libretti to her little room and we lay on our stomachs on the bed and I explained the texts of the music we had heard. I would hum it; then she would; then we would hum together. At first I took her to the lighter operas, Puccini and middle Verdi, over and over; then to the least demanding Wagner, *Die Meistersinger*. A few months later, on my birthday, she surprised me with orchestra tickets to *The Marriage of Figaro*. It was an experience actually to *sit down* at the opera.

I brought her books, a far cry from her fainting heroines: *Germinal* was the first; Dostoevski, Tolstoi, Anatole France. Schnitzler, Thomas Mann followed. Again those serious eyes. "You *are* smart," she said in a seducing voice. During the Easter vacation Anny's girl friend was away visiting her parents, and I took her place. Long after midnight we talked and made love, and we woke up happy and hungry and ate breakfast in bed, black coffee and buttered rolls (the rolls left in a basket at the door). Anny's face was as smooth as a very young girl's.

Closely associated with love in my mind is walking, an aspect of love forgotten in old age. We walked all over Vienna. We walked to Heiligenstadt and looked at the house where Beethoven had lived; we walked to God knows how many churches and listened to church music; we walked through museums by the score. We walked down narrow streets where every building was a museum piece itself. "How could I have learned all this in the two rooms at home?" Anny asked. I promised her that one day we would visit Rome, Paris, Florence, London, Venice—"together, Anny."

She was transferred from psychiatry to the medical department. The work was harder, she said, but there, in contrast to the psychiatric hospital, she saw fully recovered patients *leaving*. At this time I was studying ophthalmology. The eye hospital wasn't far from the Chvostek hospital, and we were able to meet during the day, if only for a few minutes.

I was always thinking of the future, our future. "Should we settle in the country or Vienna?" I asked her.

"Kommt Zeit bringt Rat—"

"Please be more specific."

"Look," she said, "don't make that face. We can't make plans for things that are still four or five years in the future."

"A doctor and a nurse," I said again, "could anything be more ideal? You would help me in the office, go with me on my house calls, and then we'd discuss the cases together."

"And you would wake me up in the middle of the night?"

"Be serious," I said. "You know what I mean."

"Of course I do."

"Then why hesitate?"

"I don't. But *Geduld*. Let's enjoy ourselves."

A great tradition in ophthalmology grew with the Vienna Medical School. Carl Stellwag von Carion is still remembered as the doctor who established the Stellwag sign in diagnosing toxic hyperthyroidism. Among other doctors who contributed to Viennese ophthalmology, Karl Koller occupies a prominent place; in 1884 he suggested cocaine as a local anesthetic for eye operations. (The father of cocaine anesthesia in general is Sigmund Freud.) Koller's discovery changed the whole concept of eye surgery; until then operations had been performed without anesthetics—a chilling thought.

Josef Meller was my eye professor, in appearance a typical Viennese burgher, round-faced, with frameless pince-nez. He was a perfectionist, and his perfectionist's creed required that every medical student become a fully equipped ophthalmologist. He was hated by his students as was no other of our professors. That dark room divided into cubicles—I recall it with horror. In those damned little torture chambers the eye-ground was to be explored with the ophthalmoscope. The source of light, a candle, was in one corner. The problem was to catch the light and get it through the lense into the ophthalmoscope, a terrible maneuver! Often I lost the light and couldn't even see the patient's eye, to say nothing of the eye-ground. Another time I lost the lens.

At the beginning of these miseries I seriously considered switching to another profession, which I had never thought of before, even in my lowest moments. Meller didn't trust anyone. The instructors were mere bystanders. The formidable *Herr Professor* walked tirelessly from cubicle to cubicle, muttering that our whole generation of medical students was no damn good. Often he grabbed the lens and ophthalmoscope and expelled the student from the cubicle. Fortunately it was so dark he didn't know exactly which one of us he had kicked out.

Yet I have to admit that up to this day I still have some knowledge of eye-ground examinations, and I owe it to old Meller. The ophthalmoscope has been greatly improved; the source of light is built into the machine, and the formerly heavy instrument is a small unit which you can put in your pocket. Hypertension, dia-

betes, kidney diseases, brain ailments—these and many other dis-
orders are revealed by the ophthalmoscope, which we hated and
learned to prize.

The ophthalmology examination consisted of three parts: theoretical knowledge; external eye ills; ophthalmoscopy. I passed the
first two parts; the third remained. In my cubicle an elderly man
sat blinking in the light of the candle. I smiled at him; he did not
respond. I succeeded in getting the light through the ophthalmoscope into his eye-ground. I looked and looked. I broke into a
gentle sweat. I didn't have the faintest idea what was wrong with
his eye.

I wanted to give up, when I heard the old man whisper, *"Herr
Doktor,* it's a simple case. Don't you know?"

"No."

I heard the old man's wheezy titter. *"Retino-chorioiditis,"* he
whispered.

"Are you sure?"

"Natürlich."

At that moment I heard the *Herr Professor*'s well-known short
steps. "Are you ready?" he asked me.

"Jawohl, Herr Professor."

"Go ahead."

"Retino-chorioiditis." I had never heard of the disease.

Silence. The old man and I waited, and only one of us was
fully confident.

Then, "Incredible!" I heard Meller exclaim. "My colleagues
and I have worked for months on this case, and *siehe da,* a young
good-for-nothing medical student diagnoses it like that. Congratulations!"

I passed the examination with honors. I still don't know what
that complicated eye disease really is, but I shall not forget it as
long as I live.

Pharmacology: it has often occurred to me during my forty-four years of practice that the most impressive part of medicine to the patient is the way the doctor writes his prescriptions—quite illegibly, in Latin! How can the pharmacist read those insane scribblings? I have been asked that question again and again.

In my medical-student days patent medicines were virtually unknown; the doctor prescribed the ingredients he thought would help the patient, and the longer the prescription, the better the patient liked it—or at least the higher his opinion of his doctor. I can recall a prescription written by an old country-doctor friend of mine: thirty-six items. Nowadays, writing short prescriptions for patent medicines which contain the essentials, I think rather nostalgically of the time when I used to brood and ponder what medications I would order under the famous Rx. I am still sure of one thing: those prescriptions had a powerful psychological effect on the patient as he sat in the pharmacy watching the pharmacist weigh the powders, mix them, pour the mixture into tiny bags. "One four times a day—no more and no less!" the pharmacist would say sternly, piercing the patient with eyes full of awful wisdom.

Ernst Pick, the pharmacology professor, was an enthusiastic teacher, and God knows he needed all the enthusiasm he could find in order to drill the knowledge of countless chemicals into the brains of his bored audience. Surgery, obstetrics and gynecology, medicine—all meant lively, colorful case-presentations. But pharmacology!—an enumeration of pills, pills, pills, for sleeping, for coughing, for increasing the bowel movement, for decreasing the bowel movement. And numbers, numbers, numbers—how many milligrams one must prescribe, how many centigrams! In the last row of that always half-dark auditorium I often fell asleep, to wake only when I heard the thunder of stamping feet. The hour was ended, thank God.

Pick spoke with tremendous enthusiasm of a recent discovery, insulin. Only a few years before, F. G. Banting had discovered a pancreas extract which changed the course of diabetes. The amount of sugar in the diabetic's blood actually decreased after he received an injection. But was it a cure or merely an alleviation? Pick, an optimist, believed it to be a cure. (To this day there is no cure.) His insulin lectures were highlights in the otherwise monotonous subject.

To my misfortune, Pick's attention was focused on me. A first cousin of my father was an outstanding physiologist, who became famous when he discovered the nutritional value of soy beans during World War I; the discovery came as a blessing to starving Central Europe, and the German government gave László the Iron Cross. Pick, the optimist, the enthusiast, assumed that László's genius had flown to my brow. Looking straight at me, he glowingly described the virtues of the opiates, digitalis leaves, cathartics, and so on and on, and waited for an affirmative move of mine. I would nod and smile. In later life—he died and is buried in New York—he even confused me with László, who had died in Marseille during World War II. "Well! And what's new in the soy-bean world?" he would cheerfully greet me at medical meetings and social gatherings; and again, as so many years before, I would nod and smile.

My false prestige suffered a critical blow at the pharmacology examination. I steadily confused the positions of decimal points for the minute amounts of drugs, and, as a final catastrophe, answered Pick's question about the consistency of chloral hydrate— a sleeping medication—by saying it was a liquid instead of a powder. He was speechless. But László saved me from flunking.

Dr. Körner, associate professor of medicine, was Anny's chief at the medical department. He was a specialist in metabolic diseases, and she had become one of his research associates. In addition to Sundays off, she now had one weekday free. She would sleep until ten, and we would meet at eleven. On sunny days in May we sat on a bench at the Burggarten, getting an early tan, and ate lunch at one of the countless restaurants in the inner city. She talked at length about her job. Research in metabolism was just beginning, and she found it fascinating. It included bacteriology. She injected material into the blood vessels of rabbits and mice and spoke as enthusiastically of it as Pick spoke of his drugs. Dr. Körner held weekly conferences with his whole staff, and Anny talked about these and about gram-positive and gram-negative bacilli. It enchanted me to hear her enumerate them: "The gram-positive bacilli are: strepto, pneumo, staphylo; lepra, anthrax, tbc; tetanus and diphtheria, botulinus, gas edema . . ." She counted them off on her fingers, which I would then kiss. Now she was teaching me. Up in the mountains, down by the lakes, in museums, sitting on park benches, or wandering along the city streets, I listened to research.

On one of her weekdays off, Anny wasn't at the apartment. There was a note: "I have to feed the rabbits." A bit unhappy, I went to the Café Klinik and studied hygiene. But the next Sunday she was there, dressed in her Sunday best rather than the usual dirndl. "Well, shall we walk?" she said. Her mouth quivered. We walked to our favorite bench in the Burggarten, facing the statue of the late Franz Josef in his uniform as commander-in-chief, complete with mighty saber. We looked at him; then I looked at her profile. Her lips were tightly closed.

Suddenly she turned to me. "He proposed," she said.

"Who?" I said, hardly believing my ears; it seemed to me she might have been referring to Franz Josef.

"Dr. Körner."

I stared at her. He was fifty, I knew, a confirmed bachelor. "He's twice your age."

"I told him yes."

I got up and walked out of the Burggarten and along the Ring-

strasse to the Votivpark. I looked up at the twin-towered Votivkirche. Was it really true?

The next night I found a letter on my dormitory bed.

Dearest Richilein,

It's over. I'm now *Frau Doktor* Erich
Körner. The wedding was at City Hall—Erich is a non-
believer. The witnesses were my father—you should have
seen him, dressed in the suit he wore at his wedding, now
much too tight—and Erich's assistant. After the wedding,
Erich went to the General Hospital and the chauffeur drove
me home. This letter is my first act as a married woman. Tonight we're going to Rome, where there is a biological congress. From there to Munich, Paris, London.

Dearest Richilein, I know how you must feel. I will never
forget the bench at the Burggarten and your pale face as I
told you. Now let me tell the whole story.

It happened only four days ago. I locked the laboratory at
eight, as usual, and walked down the stairs with the professor. He asked me what I was doing that night, and I said I
didn't have any special plans. If I'd have dinner with him,
he said, there were some technical details he would like to
discuss. I said all right—I swear I didn't think there was anything behind this. His BMW was waiting at the hospital, and
the chauffeur drove us to Heiligenstadt near the Beethoven
house. The professor's home is a villa with a spacious garden.
A butler opened the door, and I saw a huge entrance hall
with a chandelier. The dining room was just as impressive. It
all awed me, and I said hardly anything during dinner. The
professor didn't mention any technical details. He had two
glasses of wine, and I had one.

After dinner we went into the library and he walked up
and down, smoking his pipe. I was sitting in a leather chair,
waiting for the technical details, when he stopped walking.
"Fräulein Anny," he said, "do you want to marry me?" He
might have been asking me to inject a rabbit. But then I saw

him smile, as timidly as a boy. I couldn't answer. I remember smelling tobacco very close.

Well, Richilein, I still love you, but I also love him. The old man in the Berggasse would diagnose it as a perfect case of schizophrenia. Good-by. I have decided to be a faithful wife.

Anny

"Bullshit," said Herr Franz. *"Die Drecksau!* Money, stinking money, that's why she made up her mind. And you, twenty-four years old—you still don't understand?"

"THOU WHO RAISEST
THE POOR FROM MUD"

I was preparing for the last subject of the medical-school curriculum: hygiene. The professor, Dr. Grassberger, only recently appointed to that eminent position, had already achieved fame as the technical expert behind the Vienna health system. He had suggested a pipeline carrying water to the city from the mountains a hundred miles away. To this day the *Hochquellenwasserleitung* is the pride of Vienna, which has the freshest, healthiest, tastiest drinking water in the world—and it is ice-cold. Dr. Grassberger used to say, "The sewage works best if no one talks about it." Garbage in Vienna is stored in *Coloniakübeln*, metal containers with tightly fitted covers. On Sundays and holidays, even in the poorest sections, not one piece of garbage can be found on the sidewalks, only the gray *Coloniakübeln*, waiting for collection.

For us medical students the study of hygiene was a problem—as it has remained to this day. True, we learned about pasteurization, milk-dilution, cemeteries, cleanliness of swimming pools, and other subjects connected with public health. But beyond all this, "hygiene" was a collective name which included practically the whole range of medicine from anatomy to surgery, and even more. For instance, couldn't the question "What temperature is the best for growing mushrooms?" come up at a hygiene examination? The flunking rate was higher than in any other subject, but Dr. Grassberger was a kind man who never hurt a student's feelings when flunking him.

I remember one of the examinations, when a perspiring student was struggling to answer the intricate questions, and Grassberger asked, "How is it that it is easier to get tanned on a mountain than in a valley?"

"Because," the student replied with a thin air of confidence, "you are much nearer to the sun."

Everyone laughed; the student tried to hide under his desk. Grassberger bit his mustache. "You're Hungarian, aren't you?" he asked.

"Ja, Herr Professor."

"Do you know what day of the week it is?"

"Monday, *Herr Professor."*

"Correct. There was a Hungarian gypsy who was taken to the gallows on a Monday. 'The week is not starting too well,' he observed as they put the rope around his neck. The next time you come to take the exam, choose another day," Grassberger said gently.

His special love was history, and what a relief it was when, between the *Hochwasserleitung* and the *Coloniakübeln,* he turned to the history of old Vienna, now the most carefully looked-after city in the world—at any rate, so he said. He spoke about the dreadful past, when the creeks flowing across Vienna to the Danube were filled with filth—they are all covered now—and scavenging rats, and garbage was thrown from the windows into the narrow streets, and piled high there. These festering poisons contributed to Vienna's reputation as the city of bubonic plague. With such splendors of architecture, of music, to delight their eyes and ears, how could the burghers so totally neglect public health? The most devastating epidemic of the plague coincided with the greatest triumphs of baroque culture in the reign of Leopold I, himself a composer and generous benefactor of the arts. This was at the end of the seventeenth century. The population was decimated; there was even the threat of complete annihilation.

And a doctor came to Vienna. He was the greatest living doctor, a Belgian, Paul de Sorbait.

Grassberger was not a theatrical man, he would not dream of indulging in colorful gestures, but when he spoke of de Sorbait the lecture room became Olympus. "The savior of Vienna," he said, "taught at the highly esteemed medical school in Padua. Leopold invited him to come here not just as a teacher but as court physician. De Sorbait declined; he was perfectly happy where he was. The Emperor kept on sending couriers with more and more pressing invitations, and finally de Sorbait gave in, but with a proviso: he would be responsible only to the Emperor, independent of any intervention by the bureaucracy, which was already powerful.

"He arrived at the height of the epidemic in 1679," Grassberger continued. "This was two hundred years before science established beyond any doubt that diseases are caused by microorganisms, and yet the Plague Order de Sorbait issued might have been written by a modern scientist, because in it he established the basic weapons of fighting plague: isolation, prevention. The ill must be isolated, he said, the dead buried twelve feet deep and their bodies covered with lime. Their clothing, the very household articles, everything they left behind, must be burned and their homes fumigated with sulphuric acid.

"Of course a storm broke loose, not only among doctors, who resented the high-handed foreigner, but in the church and among the public in general. The church denounced him as a heretic: the plague had been sent by God to punish sinful Vienna. Businessmen complained that the forty-day isolation de Sorbait imposed threatened the economic life of the city; and as for the man in the street and his wife—and almost every one of them had lost a relative—they were horrified to think of burning the dear one's valuable clothes and furniture. Kick the damned foreigner out! But the damned foreigner did not retreat, and the Emperor supported him and the miracle took place: the plague abated and vanished, and beautiful Vienna was saved."

We must visit the great man's grave, Grassberger said. His tomb was in Saint Stephen's Cathedral. De Sorbait himself had written his own epitaph. A baroque jewel, the plaque was crowned by his coat of arms.

The epitaph read:

Thou who raisest the poor from mud: Psalm 112.
Paul de Sorbait, born in Belgium, rests here.
Musician, orator, philosopher, warrior, physician, professor.

Court physician, rector magnificus, beggar, nothing.
I was a musician to play life's melodies,
An orator to summarize life,
A philosopher to disdain life,
A warrior to endure hardship,
A physician to give service to mankind,
Rector magnificus to defend the university's privileges; but
      Death
Is deaf to the melodies of the musician,
The eloquence of the orator,
The reasoning of the philosopher,
The lectures of the professor,
The prescriptions of the doctor,
The authority of the rector; Death took me away.
Now I am a beggar, nothing.
Please pray for me.

I revisited Saint Stephen's after World War II. The plaque, the baroque jewel, had disappeared, blown to pieces in a bombing raid; the words remain.

During my examination Grassberger asked the expected questions about pasteurization and milk-dilution and general hygiene, and then suddenly switched to history, his love for which extended to ancient times.

"Who do you think was the greatest orator in the Roman Senate: Julius Caesar, Tacitus . . . ?"

"Cato," I said.

"Why Cato?"

"What he said was full of force, struck right to the point. *'Ceterum censeo. Cartago est delenda.'* "

Grassberger shrugged. "Who knows?" he said, and told me I had passed. It was like the sound of bells. I was an M.D.

Graduation day was June 25, 1926. The ceremonies were to begin at noon, but I was up at six. In my brand-new dark blue suit I went to the Café Klinik. The door was open, but no other patron had arrived so early. The chairs were on the tables; a cleaning woman was mopping the floor in the light of the unshaded bulb.

Someone came up to greet me. "Sit down, *Herr Doktor,*" Herr Franz said with a slight bow. He had called me *Herr Doktor* often enough before, but this time it was legitimate. Without waiting for my order, he went back to the kitchen and returned with a cup of coffee and a large piece of Gugelhupf. Also the *Neue Freie Presse.*

I sipped my coffee, ate my Gugelhupf, and read.

Mussolini was visiting Africa. Was not this a provocation directed at France? The Greek dictator Pangalos had abolished the monks' republic on Mount Athos. Professor Kraus was in Vienna to speak about his discovery of pituitrin. Sergei Eisenstein's *Potemkin* was a great artistic success. *Der Rosenkavalier* was to be performed that night with Lotte Lehmann as the *Fürstin Werdenberg.*

Herr Franz was peering over my shoulder. He cleared his throat.

"I will bet you, *Herr Doktor*, that that damn Greek Pangalos will break his neck. What a fool, to punish monks; holy water is stronger than guns. To me pituitrin doesn't make sense, but I suppose you know better; I am, after all, only a waiter. As for that ship the *Potemkin*—a damn shame. Mutiny! I was a soldier. If they'd ordered me to, I'd have shot my mother—but now, well, everything seems to be permitted. Lotte Lehmann, she's all right. I've never heard her, but people say she's good." He took off his pince-nez.

The graduation ceremonies took place at the *Zeremoniensaal* of the university. The *rector magnificus* read the Hippocratic Oath; then a proctor in medieval robes brought the scepter of the university to each candidate. I placed my right hand on it and said, *"Spondeo. . . . I swear. . . ."*

I was given my diploma. It was a parchment. I read: DOCTOR UNIVERSAE MEDICINAE NOMEN ET HONORES . . .

PNEUMOTHORAX

Wearing my brand-new dark blue suit, I traveled to my parents' home in Sauerbrunn. The trip required a full two hours because of the many bottlenecks in the narrow streets of ancient villages and hamlets, but I wouldn't have minded if it had taken three times as long. I was a doctor, riding in a big Daimler motor car, driven by a chauffeur. (The car went with Father's job; so did Herr Butschek, the driver. Usually Father was very stingy with them, but for this special occasion he had put them at my disposal). As we drove, Herr Butschek asked questions in a respectful tone regarding the practice of medicine, and it occurred to me that it shouldn't be too difficult in the immediate future to borrow the car without Father's knowledge.

On the evening of my arrival, one would have thought Sauerbrunn was celebrating some tremendous event. In fact, the local Workers' Gesangsverein was honoring me with a torchlight parade. They sang the *"Lied der Arbeit"* and other songs with tremendous enthusiasm, aided by the barrel of beer Father had contributed. In the same enthusiastic spirit their chairman, the *Bürgermeister*, made a speech celebrating me as a saintly benefactor of mankind. I remember wishing that Anny or Vera or, most of all, Liesl could be there to hear it. How wonderful if in the crowd listening to Herr Schweiger, who became steadily redder and redder in the face, I should see that very pale face, the deer-brown eyes and ash-blond hair! Herr Schweiger began to turn slightly purple, and I was afraid he would rupture a blood vessel. Fortunately, as he paused for breath, the crowd thought he had finished and cheered so much he didn't have the nerve to start up again.

Later, as I entered the Kurpark café, the gypsy band struck up the "Rákóczy March." I ordered wine for them, and they played the *"Csak egy kislány van a világon"* song, which brought back Vera and her faithlessness. I drank several glasses and ordered more for the gypsies.

> *Akácos ut ha vegigmegyek rajtad én*
> *Eszembe jut egy elmult. . . .*

The gypsies came over and played the song in my ear, their faces filled with romantic anguish. I ordered more wine, and we all drank together. After a while I found myself with their arms around my shoulders. Where was Anny, sweet, fickle Anny? Nowhere. Or, rather, with her damned professor. But she would soon find out how hollow he was. Surrounded by drunken gypsies who could hardly hold their violins, I sang in a mournful voice and must have wept, because I remember one of the gypsies offering me a huge red handkerchief as he slowly collapsed.

The sun was shining through the veranda into my bedroom. Mother was looking at me, shaking her head. "You are a doctor now," she said. "You must behave like one."

For the first time in six years there wasn't the familiar slight pressure in the pit of my stomach—no books, no exams. It was true that I felt sick, but that was from the night before. I was free. Internship at the Hospital of the City of Vienna would begin on the first of October. Three and a half months of freedom—and girls all over, local girls and girls who spent the summer with their parents at the Sauerbrunn spa, girls with dark red hair, with brown hair, with black hair, even with ash-blond hair! In the words of a popular song, *"Ob blond, ob braun, ich liebe alle Frau'n!"* Once and for all I would forget Vera and Anny and, most of all, Liesl.

A young doctor without any romantic attachments—how sweetly the girls looked into his eyes! Often when I got home the skies would be turning gray. The veranda door would open very quietly. In nightdress and robe Mother would put her finger to her lips, a gesture that meant: Don't wake up Father.

But none of the girls succeeded in banishing the memory of those others, and I began to feel tired, tired of the nightly excursions, and thoroughly accustomed to the title of doctor. I even felt tired of the beautiful summer. What had Goethe said? *"Nichts ist schwerer zu ertragen als eine Reihe von schönen Tagen.* Nothing is harder to endure than a series of beautiful days." I stayed at home at night and woke up very early, half past four or five. Father would get up at five or half past; he loved the garden, the fruit trees, the flowering bushes, the lawn, and would spend a couple of hours gardening before going to his office. I would look out at him and wonder why I felt tired—exhausted. Was the feeling a delayed effect of the final triumph of graduation?

My appetite was poor. "You eat like a bird," Mother said.

"It's only Goethe," I said.

This made no sense to her, and I had to explain. It still made no sense. "One should not speak of *enduring* beautiful days," she said. "Here, at least try a piece of Mohnstrudel."

I developed a little cough.

On the morning of September 18, for me an unforgettable date, I was shaving when I began to cough. Up came some light red blood. I looked into the mirror as though at a ghost: very pale face; the prominent facial bones seemed to stick out more than ever. I took the thermometer from the cabinet. In a few minutes it showed 38.5 degrees Celsius. Somehow I finished shaving. I was drying the razor when I coughed again and again expectorated blood. I washed the blood away, got dressed quickly, and left by the side door, so as not to have to face Mother, who was sweeping the floor in the front room.

I walked to Father's office and told him. Of course he wasn't a physician, but he had lived all his life with doctors. Half of the patients cared for by his sick-benefit board were tubercular. His ordinarily calm face changed, then became calm again. "Perhaps it's only a cold. We'll have Dr. Nindl take a look at you."

Dr. Nindl, the chief physician of the board, said what I expected him to say after he examined me—exactly what I would have said in his place: "We need some additional examinations." He and Father went into the next room; when they came out Dr. Nindl called the sanatorium at Grimmenstein. I expected this too, because, after all, hemoptysis is a sign of an advanced case of tuberculosis.

With Herr Butschek at the wheel and Mother beside me in the back seat, holding my hand as though I were six years old again and murmuring every once in a while, "It will be all right, it will be all right," the Daimler climbed the winding road up to the foothills of the Alps and higher. Early snow wreathed the pine trees, and the air was sharp. I remembered Vera's flushed face as we clambered to the top of the Schneeberg, and how cold her lips were, and how we devoured our bread and salami after we made love, and the sight of the valley floor far below.

Here was another mountaintop.

Grimmenstein was the sanatorium for department-store workers who had become tubercular. A thoroughly modern hospital, it was always full; tuberculosis was the number-one killer in those days. There would not have been a place for me so quickly if it had not been for Father's position, which also explained why the head of the sanatorium, Dr. Mändl, was waiting for us. He was only in his thirties but already had built an impressive reputation as a tuberculosis specialist. I remember him very well, his tall powerful body, his ruddy face, his manner.

After seeing Mother to a comfortable waiting room, he took me to his office and I undressed for the examination. "Breathe. Cough. Breathe. Cough." He pushed a button on his desk; a good-looking nurse came in. I remember thinking, even in my misery, Will I see her again? "Chest X ray: AP and lateral. Sputum. Sedrate," Dr. Mändl said.

Later, back in his office, I found him reading a wet chest film in the viewing box. He turned as I came in. "Sit down." I sat down. "Now, when did you first feel that something was wrong with you?"

"This morning, *Herr Primarius.*"

"And before? No weight loss, night sweats, cough—the early signs?"

"Well, yes and no."

"Typical of doctors. If a patient had missed any of these symptoms, you would have thought him an idiot, *nicht wahr?*"

"*Jawohl, Herr Primarius.*"

"Now settle down for the facts. I don't like wasting time. Can you read a chest film?"

"A bit."

"Have a look."

It was an easy case to evaluate: tuberculous tissue changes of both upper lung lobes, and a cavity the size of a walnut below the left clavicular bone.

The good-looking nurse came in with the lab results. Dr. Mändl looked at them. "The sputum positive for acid fasts. Sedimentation rate: fifty. Clear?"

Clear enough. "Yes, *Herr Primarius.*"

"Let's discuss it. After all, you're a doctor; you must have learned something in med school. First we'll try a pneumothorax.

If it works, *wir sind übers Wasser.* If there are adhesions, maybe a Jacobeus will do the trick. As *ultimum refugium,* thoracoplastic. *Verstanden?"*

"Yes, *Herr Primarius.*"

"Now go to bed."

He called Mother in. I remember her large frightened eyes. He took her hands in his and spoke in a cheerful tone, whereas with me his voice had been brusque. *"Wir werdens schon damachen,"* he assured her.

"Then may I take him home? *Gute Hausmannskost—"*

"I know you're a wonderful cook, but good meals alone won't help. Leave him to me."

We smiled at each other. She kissed me and left, and I was put to bed.

I could hear the Daimler start; I knew the sound of its engine and exhaust. Away it went, no doubt with Herr Butschek telling Mother that all would be well; after all, her son was a doctor. Through the big window I could see the mountains covered by a bluish haze. My wristwatch on the night table said six o'clock.

Tubercle bacilli; gram positive. How distinguished they looked through the microscope! I could hear Anny again: "Lepra, anthrax, TB." Where would she be now, with her professor? In Munich. Yes, first Rome, then Munich. And I was at Grimmenstein.

It was a well-defined cavity. It was my cavity.

The pneumothorax would work if the two leaves of the pleura were not glued together by adhesions. If it didn't work, there were other methods. If they all failed . . . ? But the dramatic surgical approach to tuberculosis was working wonders: pneumothorax, the insufflation of air between the leaves of the pleura; Jacobeus's operation, cutting through the nerve that supplies the diaphragm; thoracoplastic, removing the ribs above a cavity, thereby compressing the diseased lung and inhibiting the spread of the disease.

Despite these advances, the mortality rate from tuberculosis remained high. What was it Professor Tandler had said? "The notion that tuberculosis is caused by the bacilli which my distinguished colleague Koch discovered is only partially correct. One has only to consider the percentage of TB among the poor and among the rich."

The war: four years of standing in line for bread; never enough to eat. The years immediately after the war: Baden and our butcher uncle and his beef dripping; never quite enough to eat. The good Quaker ladies with their free breakfast, never quite enough. Two soft-boiled eggs at the Café Klinik, but never quite enough!

It seemed to me now that I owed my cavity to all those years of never quite enough and that in consequence there was more than a little doubt whether I would live to see my twenty-fifth birthday on February 4, four and a half months away.

I sat up. It was pitch-dark in the room, and I turned on the bedside light. "Light, light, glorious light!"—as old Professor Schaffer, histology, used to exclaim, enthusiastically waving his arms. I, former right wing of the Badner Athletic Club soccer team, had been lying in the darkness, internally groaning with self-pity. Shame!

A few days later I was wheeled into the operating room; after a local anesthetic had been administered, a needle was inserted between two ribs, and an apparatus pumped air into my chest. A chest X ray was taken; then I was wheeled back to my room. I lay waiting for the result.

Footsteps sounded outside. The door opened; Mändl's brusque voice: "All right."

Primarius Dr. Hanns Mändl! Often in my later life I wondered whether his behavior toward me was really what it should have been. Never a *"Herr Kollege"* from him; never, never my first name; never an expression of sympathy; his voice was always brusque. I remember his daily rounds: footsteps outside; door opening; the brusque voice. "How're you?" "No complaints, *Herr Primarius.*" "*Gut.*" And out he would go.

Once I had a bad headache late at night; I rang for the night nurse and asked for a few aspirin tablets. She left to get them; at least, that was what I thought. Footsteps outside; door opening; brusque voice: "You've got a headache?"

"Yes, *Herr Primarius.*"

He gave me a thorough check-up, looked into my eye-grounds, tested my reflexes. I knew he was trying to rule out a brain involvement.

Finally he straighted up. "If possible," he said (perhaps his tone was not quite so damnably brusque), "try to avoid treating doctors or their relatives. There is always trouble. Some wise man —perhaps it was Hippocrates himself—once said, 'If the patient recovers, God did it. If he dies, it was the doctor.' This applies triple strength when treating doctors." He turned to go. "As far as you're concerned, no meningitis. Aspirin." And out he went.

My outlook improved with an improved appetite, normal temperature, sedrate down to ten. The bacilli disappeared from my sputum. A panel in the door leading to the terrace was left open and, snugly tucked in, warm as toast, I would feel the keen air and listen with delight to the insane howling of the wind. On fine days I lay on the terrace: air temperature, zero; sun, hot. My face quickly tanned—a so-called "healthy tan"; elsewhere in the sanitorium people with tanned faces were slowly dying. (How is it that getting tanned on a mountaintop is easier than in a valley? Because you are closer to the sun. I laughed. Well, well! Laughter!)

September went, then October, November, December. In January I was allowed to work in the laboratory but not to eat with the other doctors in their dining room. Mändl discovered me there once. "Out! A patient is a patient."

February 4 passed without my funeral.

On March 15, Mändl called me to his office. His face was friendly, or almost. "The time of *Faulenzen* is over," he said. "The pneumothorax works. At the Krankenhaus der Stadt Wien you'll receive fillings three times a month for the next three years, *verstanden?* A few other orders: Live with moderation. *Moderation.* Alcohol, sex, smoking—in moderation! And a one-hour rest every afternoon." I still rest for one hour every afternoon.

"Thank you, *Herr Primarius.*" I bowed and walked to the door.

He called me back. "Now listen. Keep this as a rule for the rest of your life: no smooth we're-all-pals attitude with patients. A clear, impersonal attitude is the best for them and for you. They feel safe only if their doctor stays remote."

My son's middle name is Hanns. Hanns Mändl died at forty-three of a kidney ailment diagnosed too late. He neglected himself, as most doctors do.

✦ *ix* ✦

CITY HOSPITAL . . .

AND FINALLY, MARIA

After some weeks of Mother's *gute Hausmannskost* I reported at
the Hospital of the City of Vienna in May 1927 to begin my
internship. *Hofrat* Dr. Baumgarten, the medical director, took a
good look at me. "You look more like a boxing champ than a TB
patient," he said. "Pneumothorax, Mändl wrote to me. Hmmm."

He had been chief physician of the *Kaiserlich und Königlich
Kriegsmarine* at Pola on the Adriatic, where the Austro-Hungarian fleet had its main base, but his duties had been administrative
rather than medical. After the war he was called by Tandler to
Vienna to take over the administration of the city hospital. He
was a slightly built man with a mild manner but as strict in his
way as Mändl.

"A doctor must cure his illness while continuing with his profession," he went on. "And your first assignment will be Medical
Department II. Your tubercular bacilli can mix freely with those
of your patients." He smiled at his joke, and I did too.

Medical Department I was for general ailments. Medical Department II was for the tubercular: a tall building in back of a
quadrangular courtyard. As you approached it you could smell

the camphor which, besides morphine, was injected into terminal patients to alleviate their dyspnea and let them slip as peacefully as possible from this world into a better one.

Primarius Dr. Zaffron, chief of the department, a man over sixty with an uncombed beard and warm eyes, gave me a pleasant reception. I told him my story. "Well, I don't believe too much in these new ideas," he said. "But what else can we old people do but yield?"

"The pneumothorax helped me, *Herr Primarius.*"

"Mere accident," he said, and went on signing death certificates. "You'd have recovered anyway. But"—he sighed—"if you want to you can do your pneumothorax job on the patients."

It turned out to be a tough assignment. I was entrusted with a ward of a hundred, mostly in the terminal stage—drawn faces, the big eyes of the moribund, many of them young. I signed five to ten death certificates every day.

Our hospital training was different from American training, as I was to learn much later. In America you start with a year of rotating internship (in some hospitals you begin at once with specialist's training), followed by residency in a specialty. We were trained to become general practitioners. That took four years. The head of the department chose from among his house doctors one or two who he thought should become specialists. It was a great distinction to become a *"Herr Assistent,"* the chief's deputy, in which capacity you would spend four to five years. As a specialist, you were eligible to be head of a department.

I had a few chances during my training to become a *Herr Assistent*. Dr. Zaffron offered me the distinction. I had had good preliminary training at Grimmenstein, had become proficient in physical medicine, could read chest films and perform the pneumothorax. But a life of looking at tubercular patients did not attract me; a sad career, I thought. I told my chief a few months later that I was grateful but didn't feel I was ready to accept his offer. "A mistake," he said. "Tuberculosis has a bright future. Look at the turnover."

My next hospital assignment was ophthalmology: conjunctivitis, trachoma, cataracts, and no death certificates. Professor Lauber, with his immaculate snow-white beard, looked something like my old physics professor, Lecher. I was in difficulties with him very soon. He was an inveterate monarchist and, while making rounds and performing operations, often stated his regret that the old order was gone. His most moderate term for the republic was Pig Republic. I was a convinced republican, and it was hard to hold my tongue. Finally, when he came out with an especially juicy remark, I couldn't.

"The Hospital of the City of Vienna is a republican institution, permit me to observe, *Herr Professor,* governed by a Socialist administration."

With a lantern in his right hand, Lauber was looking into the eye of a postoperative patient. He turned on me. "Will you keep your mouth shut?"

"No," I said. "And if you want me to, I'll quit."

It was unheard of for a subordinate to defy his superior, and Lauber was so shocked he could not speak. His Adam's apple moved. Finally he squeaked out a few words: "We'll talk later."

I waited for that interview without pleasure; I thought it would be the end of my career, at least as an intern in the ophthalmology department. Even in republican Vienna, discipline was sacred. Days passed; I worked, went on the rounds with the professor, assisted him at operations. He said nothing about our controversy.

One month later, during a cataract operation, he stopped, lifted the scalpel, and glared at me.

"Now I've got it!" he shouted. "You want to know why I prefer the monarchy? Let me tell you! In the monarchy you knew which ass you had to kiss! In the republic there are too damn many!"

I could see how much this satisfied him. He turned back to the patient. Not another disagreeable word ever passed between us.

Sometimes even now I wake up and am amazed to find myself in bed in New York, because just a moment or two ago I was in my room at the Hospital of the City of Vienna, in the good wide bed with yellow blankets woven with figures resembling those of Greek mythology. A spacious closet, a desk with a leather-cushioned chair, and a balcony outside! Indeed our quarters were a comfortable home, separated from the rest of the hospital by a park.

At seven, an old lady with thick eyeglasses would tap on the door and politely mention that it was time to get up. Then she would put a sparkling white (no detergents, no phosphates!) doctor's uniform on the chair and leave, and I would get up and have a cold shower, which, I stoutly affirm, I *enjoyed,* and would soon be in the dining room, drinking a steaming cup of coffee and eating *Butterweckerln* while reading the morning paper. Perfect happiness! Those six long years in medical school were worth it.

But perfect happiness must be marred by something, or it would pass unnoticed. Mine was marred by the thrice-monthly pneumothorax and by the moderation Mändl had emphasized. Almost every night there was a party in the doctors' quarters—a birthday, an engagement, a promotion, and so on. If you left earlier than two, you were regarded as a killjoy. I had to leave at ten, after one drink—sometimes two drinks, but then my conscience would speak to me in Mändl's voice for the rest of the night and I would get up in the morning with an imaginary hangover.

From the eye department I went to surgery, the most strenuous work of all. Anesthesia was no independent, diversified discipline in those days, as it is now. The youngest intern would perform the weary job of dropping ether on a mask, perform it for hours. I should add that in all the years I spent at the Hospital of the City of Vienna I don't recall a single death from anesthesia. I assisted at operations day and night; a gastro-intestinal operation or the removal of a gall bladder would take three hours or even more.

And still my pneumothorax worked well. My lungs gave me no trouble until thirteen years later, when I was a doctor on the Ivory Coast.

In June 1927 I attended the graduation exercises of one of my friends. My afternoon was free, for a change. My friend's sister asked me what I was doing, and I said, "Nothing."

"Well, come along with me and we'll visit my girl friend," she said. "She doesn't live far from here."

I said yes, the first of a long history of such answers in this connection.

I knew my companion's girl friend, in a manner of speaking. Her name was Maria. She was the niece of a classmate who was one of the rare women medical students of the time. Occasionally I had called at this classmate's house and had been admitted by a rude little girl of eleven or twelve. I thought of her as rude because once, in kindly avuncular fashion, I offered to help her with the homework which obviously was causing her great pain, and she stuck out her tongue at me. After that I left her strictly alone and as a matter of fact soon stopped calling at her aunt's apartment.

This afternoon the same archaic elevator carried us inch by inch to the top floor. The elevator was even slower than I remembered, but of course it was five or six years older. My companion knocked on the apartment door, and presently a girl opened it. She wore a dirndl with a white apron. Her face was lightly tanned. Her hair was darkish blond. She wore a trace of lipstick.

She was stunning.

I looked at her in silence as she greeted my companion. Then she looked at me and spoke. "Haven't we met somewhere?"

"Once upon a time," I said, "I offered to help you with your homework."

She pursed her lips. "Ah, so that was you."

"I'm afraid so," I said.

"Why afraid?"

"Because you didn't like me."

"That's true," she said. "I didn't."

"Have things changed?" I asked humorously.

"No."

The two girls burst into laughter and proceeded to talk about a multitude of trivial things in quick voices. I withdrew to a corner. After a while it seemed to me I had better withdraw altogether, and I got up and moved toward the door.

"Are you going already?" Maria asked.

"I don't like to interfere," I said.

This must have dimly stirred her conscience. "We're going across the street to have some ice cream. Why don't you come with us?"

"Are you sure I won't be interfering?"

She smiled.

So we went across the street for ice cream, and the two girls continued to talk. By and by my friend's sister looked at her watch, said she was late for an engagement, and left. Maria and I were alone.

"More ice cream?" I said.

"No, thank you. You sound angry."

"I am."

"Why?"

"I can only say you haven't changed much—I mean temperamentally."

She smiled again. "It's stuffy in here, isn't it? Why don't we go for a walk?"

We walked to the nearby Augarten and sat on a bench. How often I had sat on park benches with Vera and Anny! Maria asked politely, as though to make amends, if I wouldn't tell her something about my current activities, so I told her about the hospital. She smiled politely throughout, and I thought the thought that had struck me when she opened the door: She was stunning.

But she was much too young for me. I was, after all, twenty-five.

"Must get back to work, I'm afraid," I said. "Well, I hope we'll meet again."

"It wouldn't make too much sense," she said. "I'm just about to get engaged."

"What a coincidence!" I exclaimed. "I am too!"

I walked her home. We parted coolly.

Jacob Erdheim, head of the pathology department, stood out among the professors at the hospital. His reputation was world-wide; two generations of American doctors had come to Vienna for postgraduate training under him, and I am sure they remember him as I do, vividly.

He was remarkable in many ways. Very tall and thin, he had a boy's piping voice. In fact he was a eunuch. He lived at the hospital in one of the meanest rooms, by choice; he could have had a suite. I don't believe his pale, long face ever felt the sun. He walked from his cheerless room to the dining room for breakfast, then to his department, back to the dining room for lunch, back to his department, back to the dining room for dinner, back to his department, and eventually back to bed—day after day after day, year after year after year.

We looked at him with respect, but if there was anyone in the whole hospital who added to it a touch of friendliness, I don't know who it could have been. He was a terror not only to us low-ranking doctors but to department heads. In Vienna every patient who died in a hospital was given a post mortem. The operation was performed at seven in the morning, and from the profes-

sors down to the newest intern we trembled when Erdheim began
his work. Had we—the person involved—made the right diagnosis? The post mortem would prove us right or wrong. I have seen
a gray-haired professor, an eminent man, stand blushing and
trembling like a schoolboy as Erdheim pronounced his verdict.
"Ja, Herr Kollege," the incongruous piping voice would say, "no
pneumonia! Would you care to look, *bitte?* A nice little lung
cancer, isn't it?"

Then, as happens to this very day, the buck was passed from
the top of the ladder down to the newest intern. Had the patient's history been taken with proper care? Had lab tests been
evaluated correctly? What about the X rays? The hour following
the post mortems was pure torture.

The worst errors were committed in Medical Department I, the
department for internal medicine; in the surgical departments
the diagnosis was verified at the operation ("the only discipline
in medicine which you can *grasp,*" as Billroth had said). How
well I remember Erdheim's cold eye turning from cold body to
warmly blushing professor or intern—or me. *"Ja, Herr Kollege . . ."*

The Erdheim tumors, cystic growths at the base of the skull,
were his discovery, and he was one of the first pathologists to recognize the clinical importance of the coronary arteries.

Father was away, attending an international conference on Social Security in Berlin, and the official Daimler rested peacefully
in the garage. I spent the weekend at Sauerbrunn. Again Herr
Butschek made some observations and asked my opinion of this
and that. In return I asked him for the car keys. A shadow crossed
his brow. I took out a five-schilling note. It disappeared; in its
place, lo, there were the car keys.

On Sunday morning I drove to Vienna, drove around aimlessly, looked at girls walking with boy friends, at lovers clasped
on park benches, at statues, and so on. I thought of ash-blond

hair. I thought of slightly darker blond hair and suddenly found myself in the street where Maria lived.

Well, perhaps she would like to drive around a little. The groaning elevator carried me aloft. I knocked on the door, but there was no answer. I wrote a note, slipped it under the door: "Sorry to find no one home, R. Berczeller."

A few days later I had a phone call at the hospital, a voice I didn't recognize. "So sorry I wasn't home when you called."

Maria.

"Well, I happened to have my father's Daimler, and I thought you might like to take a little drive."

"Oh, I *am* sorry."

"Perhaps some other time?"

"I don't know. Let me think it over. Good-by for now."

"Wait a minute," I said. "What about July fifteenth, at three? I'll be off that afternoon, with Father's car."

"All right," she said crisply. "One block from our house, at the Donaukanal." And bang went the receiver. What a temperament!

The Daimler was the only reason she gave in, I felt sure.

On July 15 there was a revolution in Vienna. The workers set the Palace of Justice on fire. The police intervened, and finally the Army. Gunfire followed. Eighty-five people were killed and thousands wounded. At the City Hospital we worked around the clock. I forgot all about Maria.

The revolution wasn't the only reason. I was working in Medical Department I, and the chief asked me if I would be interested in becoming a specialist in internal medicine. This was a great distinction, and I said yes at once. But it meant even more work: attending rounds, supervising the histories and physicals, and reading, reading, reading.

Sometimes I staggered rather than walked from ward to ward and didn't go home for weekends. Mother came for a visit. "You always have to go to extremes," she said, "driving yourself to the

limit. The little bit of extra flesh you gained at Grimmenstein—
where is it?" She gave me the cake she had brought, and I promised to be more careful.

Winter passed, and the spring. One night I went to a colleague's wedding party—a garden party, as it happened, with lots
of guests, wine and Schnaps, a dance band. I sat in a corner, dealing very slowly with my first drink, since it would have to last a
long time; although perhaps tonight I'd permit myself a second,
around midnight. Also very slowly I smoked one of the half-dozen
cigarettes that were my daily ration. I watched the dancers. And
there was Maria, dancing with a tall good-looking fourth-year
medical student who practiced under my supervision. He saw me,
nodded with a smile, and whispered something in Maria's ear.
She turned toward me.

She was wearing a blue sweater and short pleated skirt, very
informal for a wedding party and also very becoming. Her dark
blond hair hung loosely down to her shoulders. Today I can hum
the tune the band was playing, an English waltz.

I waved to the handsome couple, smiled, sipped my drink,
smoked my cigarette, and with half-closed eyes watched them
through the smoke.

When the waltz ended they came over. *"Herr Doktor,* my
fiancée," he said.

"We know each other, don't we?" I said.

She nodded. "Yes indeed."

"Oh? Is that so?" he said.

"Very casually," Maria said.

"We're getting married as soon as I graduate," he said.

"I congratulate you," I said.

The band struck up a fox trot. Off they went. I lit another
cigarette. She was more stunning than ever. By now she was certainly at least eighteen, very much a young lady—and quick-
tempered and arrogant, I thought; also, engaged. Forget it.

Very well! No sooner said than done. She was forgotten.

The next day, after a lot of trouble, I managed to get her on the phone. I was only calling, I said, to explain about the engagement I had broken last July 15, because of circumstances beyond my control, the revolution. "Is there always a revolution or something when you don't show up for a date?" she asked.

"Let's meet somewhere and have a nice talk," I suggested.

"No," she said.

"I would like to make up for July fifteenth."

"You would like to make up for it by having a nice talk! How conceited you are. You should have seen yourself last night, sitting in that corner like a Turkish potentate."

"Like a Turkish potentate?" I said.

"With your half-lidded eyes, smoking and sneering."

"I was not sneering."

"Kindly don't correct me with your Burgenland accent. Am I supposed to sink at your feet like a Caucasian slave or something? '*Ja, Herr Doktor, danke, Herr Doktor,* when can we meet, please?'"

I almost hung up but did not. "Please," I said.

A long silence. Suddenly her voice: "Where and when?"

"Tomorrow at four at Hüsbner's Kursalon."

"Tomorrow," she said, "just happens to be another July fifteenth."

"The Palace of Justice is not set on fire every July fifteenth."

She laughed. "All right!"

That night several patients died, there were a lot of emergency admissions, and I didn't get to bed at all. The morning was filled with work. It was half past twelve when I fell on my bed, after asking the switchboard operator to be sure to call me at three. When I woke up it was four. I didn't have time to denounce the operator—who, I learned later, had rung and rung—didn't have time to shave, almost fractured my legs getting into my trousers. I ran to a taxi I saw at the corner, yelled at the driver to rush to the café—double fare if he drove at double speed. He did, but even so it was quarter to five.

Of course she was not there. I sat down and ordered a double Cognac.

A stunning girl in a blue dress and wide gray felt hat came through the door and approached me with a smile. "I am so sorry," she said sweetly. "I couldn't get a cab, and the damned streetcar took forever."

"Are you in love with Ernst?" I said. I was somewhat light-headed from lack of sleep, running, the double Cognac, and the sight of her.

"What do you mean?"

"You can't be really in love with him," I said, "not the way we are with each other."

After several more meetings we decided that we would get married as soon as I was promoted to *Herr Assistent,* with a salary of four hundred and ten schillings and an apartment at the hospital.

That was not to be for some time.

$\ll$ { $\mathcal{X}$ } $\gg$

CHRISTMAS 1928

When Christmas of 1928 arrived, I was the youngest resident of the Medical Department in the Hospital of the City of Vienna, and it was not surprising that my seniors should elect me to remain behind while they went off to enjoy the two-day Austrian Christmas. For the first time I was to have the responsibility of the entire department, with its 250 patients, and naturally I was frightened. Again and again I heard the old proverb that plunging into deep water was the quickest way to learn how to swim.

On Christmas Eve my colleagues left, one by one. Earlier, the chief resident had made the afternoon rounds with me to discuss the most important cases. He was already in his ski clothes.

"Don't worry, Richard." He waved agreeably. "I have confidence in you. New admissions are rare during holidays, and if by chance you find yourself in trouble, you can always look things up in the Schnirer." *Medizinal-Index und Therapeutisches Vademecum,* by a Dr. Schnirer, was a popular medical pocket-manual used by generations of Viennese doctors.

We returned to the *Dienstzimmer*—the doctors' quarters—on the third floor, where the chief resident picked up his skis. He

would spend the Christmas holiday on the Hohe Wand, a moun‑
tain near Vienna. Before departing, he paused in the doorway for
a final word. I waited attentively.

"Cheer up, Richard," he said. Then he was off.

From the window I watched him leave the building, his skis
slung over his shoulders. There was no doubt now; I was really in
charge. My feeling of abandonment was intensified by the curtain
of falling snow which all but obscured the buildings across the
quadrangle. It had been storming intermittently for several
weeks, and snow had drifted in places, to make a small range of
mountains. The Hospital of the City of Vienna, popularly called
Jubiläumsspital, since it was erected during the sixtieth anniver‑
sary of the reign of Emperor Franz Josef, was situated in what was
then open country, an hour's trip by trolley from the center of the
metropolis. The city fathers had meant well, building their hos‑
pital far from smoky chimneypots and factories; and, true
enough, spring, summer, and autumn were beautiful in that sub‑
urb, especially with the nearby expanse of the old Tiergarten.
But winter was harsh, and the hospital was often virtually iso‑
lated from the rest of the world. It was difficult to walk from one
hospital department to another, or to the dining room, which was
located in a separate building. Winter of 1928 was one of the
worst in memory, and the Christmas holidays were the worst of
the season.

Night fell early that Christmas Eve. In the *Tagraum*—the large
social room—a mammoth fir tree rose almost to the high ceiling.
For several days the patients had helped the Sisters of Charity,
who served as nurses, to decorate it with tiny doughnuts, oranges,
figs, dates, candies, and chocolate bars, all wrapped in multicol‑
ored tissue. Now it stood gleaming with a hundred candles—red,
green, yellow. *"Stille Nacht, Heilige Nacht"* sounded through the
corridors, and sisters and patients assembled around the tree to
pray before dispersing to their sickrooms.

My evening rounds were about to begin. I set off for the ward where the most serious cases were confined. Sister Pia, the head nurse, awaited me with chart-book in hand. She was an elderly woman with a frail, marble-white face and pale blue eyes, always half closed behind her silver-rimmed spectacles. She was the power behind the throne in our department. Even our chief, a high-ranking internist, would never disregard an opinion pronounced by Sister Pia. She spoke softly, in the dialect of her Sudeten German homeland, and a slight lifting of her head sufficed to stifle any opposition. We young doctors were seldom addressed by her.

I approached her diffidently. She wished me a good evening and without hesitation turned to lead the way to our first patient. He was a young man in an advanced stage of pneumonia, one of many similar cases in the ward. In those days pneumonia was the principal cause of death among the acutely ill. As I adjusted my stethoscope, I saw to my embarrassment that my hand was shaking. A short time later Sister Pia leaned toward me and said in her prayer whisper, "Don't be afraid, *Herr Doktor*. I remember many, many young doctors in these past forty years who were not so sure of themselves when they started out. Now they are old professors with long gray beards." She lifted her thin brows and with fragile fingers stroked an imaginary beard. I took a deep breath.

As we walked from bed to bed, Sister Pia made notes and occasionally whispered advice. We continued through the remaining wards until she warned me that it was nearly eight o'clock, when the dining room would close. I could hardly believe that I had already survived several hours.

"Don't rush through your supper," said Sister Pia. "There's a long night ahead."

After dressing in my heavy boots and overcoat for the short trip to the dining room—I would not wear a hat under any circumstances, depending on my thick crop of hair to protect me—I pushed out into the snow, which seemed to be falling faster. Perhaps none of my colleagues would be able to return, I thought despondently. In the dining room only one of the three waitresses was on hand to serve during the holidays. Like me, she was the youngest and had been left behind. She was in a peevish mood and looked pointedly at the clock.

"It's Christmas Eve," she said, "and I also would like to be with my family."

I promised to eat as quickly as possible, and she grudgingly brought the first course, a bowl of chicken soup. As I began to spoon it the telephone rang. The waitress answered it and nodded toward me.

The admitting physician, Dr. Kreisler, was on the other end of the wire. "Sorry," he said, "I know you must be eating. Well, an ambulance is on its way with a morphine-poisoning case. Better come over and take a look."

I gestured helplessly at the waitress and climbed back into my arctic gear. I had not yet reached the door when the phone rang again, and again it was Kreisler.

"Stay there. The man died on his way here. The ambulance doctor asked if he could leave the corpse in our morgue. I said yes. Do you know the rules? I don't, and I couldn't find anybody in at the office. Anyway, tomorrow a relative or friend, if he has any, will arrange to have the body picked up. Maybe we'll have a *stille Nacht* yet."

My soup had cooled off and was taken back to the kitchen to be reheated. The heavenly scent of *Weihnachtskuchen* wafted through the room as the kitchen door opened, and my hunger had become quite painful by the time the waitress returned. The minute she placed the bowl before me the telephone rang. I did not dare look at her. This time I listened to a throaty voice with a heavy Viennese accent, the night watchman.

"Come as fast as you can," he said.

"What's wrong?"

"He's alive."

"Who?"

"The dead man. After the ambulance leaves, I lock the door from the outside—it's the rule. Suddenly I hear a groan. Where does it come from? I ask myself. I listen again. Now I hear a bump. Well, I think, what goes on in there? I go in, and, *Herr Doktor*, I can hardly believe my eyes. The corpse on the table has turned over, and one eye is squinting!"

I wondered, was Herr Hasenbichler sober? One met him at night while he walked his rounds, nodding his head, a lantern dangling from a soldier's belt. In his old, faded uniform, decorated with a medal earned in one of the earlier wars of the Habsburg Empire, he would have made an ideal poster for any veterans' organization. But the watchman was known to like his glass of Schnaps. Who would deny him an extra glass or so on Christmas Eve? I phoned Kreisler for advice.

"Don't be a fool, Richard." He laughed. "Hasenbichler—that old *Frosch!* Look, the ambulance doctor told me he found twenty empty two-c.c. ampoules of morphine on the patient's night table, and an empty syringe. Forget it."

Kreisler was a senior resident, but still . . . Improbable as Hasenbichler's account was, I could not afford to ignore it.

"Please," I said to the waitress, "five minutes more. I'm sure it's a false alarm."

I dressed rapidly and pushed through the snow the three hundred yards to the morgue, arriving, quite winded, just in time to find Hasenbichler locking the door.

"Too late," he said.

So, I thought, I had fallen for his story. I would be the laughingstock of the hospital.

"He is on his stomach all right," Hasenbichler continued, "and the blanket has fallen to the floor. Suddenly he moans and gasps, like this—ahhhh. Now he's *really* dead."

"Unlock the door," I said sharply. The old soldier obeyed in an instant.

The morgue was dimly lighted. Several corpses lay on dissection tables, covered by linen. I followed Hasenbichler to a table where a man in a white cotton shirt and wrinkled khaki trousers lay—on his stomach.

"Wasn't he on his stomach to begin with?" I said rather sternly.

Hasenbichler slowly shook his head. "No, *Herr Doktor.*"

"Let's turn him over," I said.

His arms fell limp as we did so. I switched on my flashlight and lifted the man's eyelids. His pupils were dots. With a start I thought, The pupils of the dead are dilated to a maximum. But it was no use. When I applied my stethoscope to the man's chest, I could hear nothing.

I held the stethoscope in place while I tried to puzzle out the contradiction. Suddenly I heard a faint beat, like rain striking a distant windowpane. There was a long pause, and then it was repeated. Was I hallucinating? I looked at Herr Hasenbichler. He stood motionless, his lower lip touching his mustache. I glanced around the whitewashed walls and up at the ceiling. Nothing moved. I held my breath. I could hear my own heartbeat. Was it that? I placed the stethoscope again on the man's chest. Now I heard it distinctly—a beat, a pause, a beat. I timed the beats: only ten in one minute. Six seconds between beats; it seemed impossible.

I took a mirror from my pocket and put it at the man's mouth. When I removed it, I must have shouted. Hasenbichler jumped. *"Was is denn los?"* he said.

I showed him the mist covering the mirror. At the same moment I felt triumph and panic. What was to be done next? If I called the department, it would take the stretcher-bearers ten minutes to reach the morgue and another ten to return to the hospital. Obviously treatment had to begin at once. But I had never before been confronted with a case of morphine poisoning.

Then I thought of the Schnirer in my pocket. I turned to the chapter on opium poisoning and read:

> Opium and its derivatives depress the respiratory center. The pupils are the size of pinpoints and do not react to light and accommodation. The main symptoms are drowsiness, leading to deep sleep, quasi-unconsciousness, and finally death through paralysis of the respiratory center. Continuous reflex stimulation—slapping, pinching, shaking—can revive the center. Artificial respiration is imperative as first aid. Oxygen and caffeine are the methods of choice.

I also read that the respiratory rate in such cases could diminish to as little as six breaths per minute, and that the heart rate slowed down accordingly. Was it possible that so sluggish an action could carry enough blood to the heart to keep it beating? I looked up and met Hasenbichler's little eyes embedded in a thousand tiny wrinkles. You arrogant chap, he seemed to be thinking, you thought you knew everything.

"Give me a hand," I said.

We lifted the man down to the floor. I immediately started artificial respiration with one hand, and with the other I slapped and pinched the man's face. Hasenbichler coughed to catch my attention and said, "Excuse me, *Herr Doktor,* allow me . . ."

I stood up. With hands as big as shovels, Hasenbichler seized the patient's arms, lifted them high, and then dashed them down to the man's chest, almost crushing it. I watched in wonder. It had sounded much easier in the Schnirer. The man's color remained gray. After a time, I saw large pearls of perspiration running down Hasenbichler's face. Reluctantly he turned the patient over to me for a short while, and then he resumed.

Eventually I discovered a slight change in the patient's complexion, which began to show a faint flush of pink that gradually deepened. I at once started to pinch and slap his cheeks. Suddenly a deep sigh came from the man, and his chest began visibly moving in and out. I ran to the phone and called my department, asking for Sister Pia.

"Thank heavens," she said. "There you are. It's after midnight."

I told her the story, trying to conceal my elation. I had indeed jumped into deep water and learned how to swim.

"For pity's sake," she said when I finished, her voice rising ever so slightly. "Why didn't you call me at once? The man needs oxygen and more oxygen and caffeine. But, *Herr Doktor* Berczeller, we are in a hospital!"

I stuttered an apology.

"Never mind," said Sister Pia, once more composed. "The man is alive, and that's all that matters. I'll send a stretcher."

When I returned to the patient, he had just opened his eyes. They were bloodshot and fluttered with the effort of accommodating light. His face was puffed and his lips were swollen.

"Leave me alone, please," he whispered.

"No, sir," said Hasenbichler at my side. "You don't make a fool of me a second time."

Nevertheless the patient closed his eyes. His breathing instantly diminished. I shook him, and he looked up again.

"You must stay awake," I said.

Two attendants arrived with a stretcher, and only when the patient had been placed on it did I realize he was an exceptionally tall man, probably three or four inches over six feet. Fortunately for the bearers, he was also slender. We made a strange procession through the snow—the stretcher first, followed by Hasenbichler, holding aloft his lantern, and me.

"Herr Hasenbichler," I said, "how do you feel after saving a human life?"

He chuckled with embarrassment. "Morphine, imagine! How the world has changed. In the old days fancy people used the shotgun. Do you remember Crown Prince Rudolf and the Vetsera? How could you? You were not even born. Poor people, of course, used the rope. And young maids in lovers' grief drank lye. I remember a girl . . . Well, it was long ago."

At the hospital door he said good night. I saw his lantern bobbing through the snowfall as he resumed his rounds.

The stretcher barely fitted into the old elevator. It was one of those archaic cagelike structures, which projected from the wall. From the ground floor one could see the moving loops of cable and the jerking ascent of the car. There wasn't room for me, so I walked up the three flights of stairs beside the shaft, nearly keeping pace with the car. Sister Pia was waiting at the elevator door, and the patient was swiftly carried to a bed made up in the *Tagraum*.

"Is this the only space we have?" I asked timidly.

"It's better here," she said. "There will be a lot of activity, and why disturb the other patients, *Herr Doktor?*" She immediately strapped an oxygen mask around the patient's mouth and handed me a syringe filled with caffeine. The patient had again lapsed into unconsciousness, and I began to think that Hasenbichler's gymnastics might have been in vain. But the oxygen and the stimulant worked with surprising speed. In fifteen minutes the patient reopened his eyes. Meanwhile Sister Pia questioned me closely about the episode in the morgue.

"What do you suppose happened?" she asked. "A man in his condition doesn't spring to life."

"I don't know," I said. "According to Hasenbichler, he was just lying there."

"Those ambulance men, I suppose," she whispered. "They handle the dead like sacks of potatoes. They probably threw our giant on a table, and it must have produced the reflex stimulation to his respiratory center, no?"

I nodded my head, astonished. I had never thought of that possibility.

The sister's prominent nasolabial folds smoothed out—as close as she could come to a smile.

We still had many other patients on the critical list to attend to, and after putting a nurse in charge of the morphinist, Sister Pia led the way to the wards with a lift of her sea-gull hat.

When we returned to the *Tagraum,* our patient was fighting the nurse, who was trying to keep the oxygen mask over his mouth. He was without doubt very much alive. His eyes looked clearer to me, and I decided to experiment by withholding the oxygen. He continued breathing evenly, and his pulse had increased to fifty beats a minute. He still had difficulty accommodating even the weak light in the room and squinted repeatedly. Each time he closed his eyes I shook him, a sequence that became routine for the next hour. He would look straight into my face and mutter, "Leave me alone, *Herr Doktor.*" Even these few words were enough to reveal a refined German used by upper-class Viennese.

Now that his appearance was returning to normal, I could see that he was a handsome man, about fifty, with thick graying hair and an oval face. Sister Pia was observing him closely too, waiting for the moment when she could get information for the admissions office. Finally he seemed sufficiently awake to communicate, and she said she must ask him a few questions.

He turned away from her. "Must it be?" he asked mournfully.

"Yes," she answered. "Your name, please."

There was a pause, and then he said, "Bauer . . . Alfred."

"Your age and occupation?"

"Please, Sister . . ."

Sister Pia pressed the chart to her chest. "We have our rules, Herr Bauer," she said. "Four hours, at the latest, after admission we must have personal data—although we must admit you are here under somewhat unusual circumstances."

I suppressed a smile but saw that she did not intend humor.

"You must stay alive. God gave you life, and you should be grateful," she continued, lifting her brows.

"All right," he said wearily. "I'm an electrical engineer . . . if

I find a job . . . I'm fifty-five . . . I live alone . . . I'm single
. . . my nearest relative is a cousin who lives in Linz. Now may
I rest, please?"

At this point I took over for an examination He could sit up
without help, and, apart from the effect of the drug, he was in
perfect physical health. I noted a large scar with irregular edges
on the upper part of his abdomen. It looked to me like the mark
of dum-dum bullets often seen on the wounded of World War I. I
touched it with my finger.

"It's old, *Herr Doktor*. What does it matter?" Bauer said.

I continued to make notes on the chart. "Do you use morphine
habitually?" I asked. "Was it an accidental overdose, or did
you . . ."

Bauer had closed his eyes. I shook him.

"Doctor, are you a gentleman?" he said.

"You must stay awake."

"A gentleman minds his own business."

Sister Pia whispered into my ear, "It's enough for the time
being."

It was two o'clock. In the quiet, one heard only the shuffling
steps of the patients walking to and from the lavatories. Suddenly
I felt very tired.

"Herr Bauer," I said, "you must stay awake. It will be better
for both of us. Let's talk. What are you interested in? Politics?
Music? Art?"

"I am interested in nothing."

"All right," I said. I had read in my Schnirer that the peripa-
tetic method could be used to foster circulation. (This has long
since been abandoned in the medical profession, because in fact it
is supposed to cause a drop in blood pressure.) "We're going to
take you for a walk."

After the expected protest, Bauer stepped down from his bed.
He was indeed a giant, almost a head taller than I, and Sister Pia,
who supported his first steps, looked like a tiny child.

"What a pity," she said, looking up at him as though he were a tree.

We began our promenade around the room, walking first in one direction and then in the other. I now understood why the remarkable Sister Pia had prepared the bed in the *Tagraum*. I told medical anecdotes and tried to interest Bauer in the doctor's problems of keeping people alive. I don't know how long our marathon went on, but suddenly I could not walk another step. Still the patient had to be kept occupied. I thought of a card game.

Sister Pia produced a pack of cards from a cabinet, and I sat down at a table, inviting Bauer to take the seat opposite.

"What will you have," I asked, shuffling the cards. *"Einundzwanzig?* Meriasch?"

He chose Meriasch. I cut the cards and dealt. After a few plays, I discovered that Bauer was trying to nap behind his cards.

"Would you rather walk?" I asked in warning.

Little by little his interest grew, at least enough to have a reasonably intelligent game, although occasionally when he lifted a card to make a play, his hand would freeze in midair. I would wake him and review the play just made, and the game would continue. I also tried to get more data on him.

"How did you get onto morphine?" I asked.

He was shuffling cards. He looked at me in surprise. "You saw the scar. I spent most of the war in hospitals. I got lots of morphine. After the war I used it off and on, mostly when there was trouble. I was in and out of jobs—you know."

"And the trouble this time? A woman?"

"Oh, no. Why do you want a reason? Must there be a reason? Don't you believe a man can wake up one day and decide he's had enough?"

He became agitated, dealt too many cards, and had to begin again. To restore his humor, I suggested we bet a groschen a play. He took this up, played with great intensity, and won thirty hands in a row. By this time I had grown so tired I could hardly concentrate, and my forgotten hunger was again burning into my stomach. I recall looking at the darkened corner where the Christmas tree stood, and the next thing I knew, someone was shaking my shoulder. I looked up into the smiling face of Bauer.

"Your move, Doctor," he said.

Meanwhile Sister Pia had been coming and going quietly. She stopped in front of me.

"Doctor," she said, "take a brief rest, even for half an hour."

"Good idea," said Bauer, collecting the cards.

I knew that I should stay at my post; I was responsible for everything. And yet, if only I could close my eyes for a few minutes . . .

"I'll keep an eye on things," Sister Pia assured me.

I gave a final, appraising look at Bauer. Then I staggered off to the *Dienstzimmer.* There I collapsed, fully clothed, on the bed and passed immediately into a deep slumber.

House doctors sleep with one ear open. Through my dreams I heard a distant crash. Shortly afterward, someone opened the door to my room. Peering through the slits of my eyes, I saw first a burning candle and then the pale face of Sister Pia.

"Doctor," she whispered, "the morphinist."

I leaped up. Sister Pia accompanied me to the *Tagraum,* where patients stood around in their hospital robes, waiting, apparently wakened by the crash. Early daylight showed through the window. The morphinist's bed was empty.

"Where is he?" I asked.

"There," said Sister Pia, leading me to the staircase. "He broke away."

The space between the staircase and the elevator formed a wide shaft. I looked into its depth and saw sprawled at the bottom a man's figure. Slowly I began to descend the stairs.

"Do you need me?" asked Sister Pia.

"No," I said.

I shuddered in anticipation of the bloody, fractured body of
the morphinist. By the time I reached the bottom of the stairs, I
had involuntarily closed my eyes. When I opened them, I was
relieved to see that this was a tidy suicide after all. There was no
blood in sight. The body lay on its stomach, the head turned to
one side. I walked up to it. The limbs seemed in normal position,
and, as a matter of fact, the facial complexion looked healthier
than before. I leaned down. The morphinist was snoring peacefully.

I slapped him smartly on the face. At once he rolled over,
stretched his arms, and yawned. At the same instant I heard a
rustling behind me and turned to see Herr Hasenbichler struggling up from a kneeling position. With one hand he held his hat
and with the other he scratched his bald head.

"Lately one cannot be sure of one's life," he moaned. "I came
in on my morning rounds—it's the rule," he said, "—and suddenly I feel something heavy falling on my back—not my back,
but here." He indicated his right hip. *"Der Strolch*—why is he
picking on me?"

"For God's sake," I said, "are you all in one piece?"

"Yes," he said, "but my lantern . . ."

The lantern was indeed damaged, the glass broken and the entire metal frame bent. I assured him that he would be issued another, just as good. I returned to Bauer, who was now snoring on
his back. After examining him quickly for fractures, I asked him
in a firm voice to wake up. He opened his eyes and said, "Did you
have a nice rest?"

I did not reply but commanded him to precede me up the
stairs. He obeyed without protest. When we entered the *Tagraum,* we saw Sister Pia kneeling at the tree. She finished her
prayer, made a sign of the cross in slow motion, and rose. She
looked very much shaken. Advancing almost timidly, she studied
Bauer from head to toe.

"Merry Christmas," he said, bowing.

I recalled a bed in the storeroom, an old structure with a high railing around it, once probably used for psychiatric patients. I ordered it moved to a private room and took Bauer there under the escort of two attendants. I had not spoken to him since his second resurrection.

"Why are you angry?" he asked. At first he thought the bed was a joke, but eventually he crawled into it. The railing was equipped with a lock, which I secured.

"You don't have much confidence in me," he complained.

I couldn't help smiling. Before I left, I pressed thirty groschen —the money he had won in the card game—into his hand.

In the *Tagraum*, Sister Pia was waiting to begin our morning rounds. She was quite recovered, standing erect, her sea-gull hat crisp and pert, the chart-book pressed to her bosom.

The morphinist was discharged two days after Christmas. For several weeks I searched for his name in the daily obituaries. He never came back. As for me, when I appeared at breakfast after the holidays, my colleagues greeted me with cheers.

⚜{ XI }⚜

PATERNITY

The reason for the long delay before Maria and I could get married was the death in November 1929 of old Dr. Klinger in Mattersburg, a town of four thousand or so in Burgenland, a few kilometers from the city where I had grown up—and contracted the accent Maria had referred to. He had been the town's Jewish doctor for more than fifty years. The only other doctor, the gentile doctor, could not possibly provide sufficient medical care for Mattersburg and the surrounding villages and hamlets strewn all over the Rosalia Mountains, and I felt a strong urge to take Dr. Klinger's place.

I was well into my training as a *Herr Assistent,* and I had an agreeable relationship with my chief. Why should I want to exchange the amenities of Vienna for a life in the woods? Nevertheless, my urge grew stronger. I remembered how beautiful Burgenland was, and I recalled Dr. Klinger's house in the center of town, a spacious two-story building painted egg-yellow, with a large courtyard shaded by walnut trees.

Maria's grandmother, with whom she lived, since her mother was dead, had asked us to wait for a year before "rushing into marriage," and in any case a hospital apartment would not be available for a while. I spoke enthusiastically to Maria about the enormous services a doctor can perform for country people. She said I was running after a childhood dream.

"Let me run just for a little," I said.

Finally I compromised and asked my chief for a half-year's leave of absence. With some reluctance, protesting that it was not really in my best interests, he granted it, and I went down to Mattersburg to visit Frau Klinger.

I had thought of renting Dr. Klinger's old office and a couple of rooms in the spacious yellow house, but Frau Klinger told me regretfully that she preferred to live her remaining years alone in the house. I walked streeet after street, looking for suitable quarters in which to set up my practice. The ghetto had remained unchanged for centuries. Among the many buildings in the main square I discovered a two-story building with a grocery store on the first floor and an apartment above. It was a modern apartment by Mattersburg standards, and I took it at once, paying four months' rent in advance. Then I telephoned Maria.

The day my black nameplate, lettered in gold, was nailed on the entrance door, snow fell mixed with icy rain, but my heart felt as if it were spring. Upstairs, I had divided the apartment into office and living quarters. The office was equipped with the most modern tools and instruments, which I had arranged neatly in gray cabinets, and in a corner stood my X-ray machine. It was certainly the only one in a Burgenland doctor's office. Out in front of the building waited my little Opel-Steyr, which I had bought on the installment plan—as I had bought everything else. I was ready to receive patients and to make house calls.

No one came on the first day, or the day after. I was not worried; people must be given time to learn about the arrival of a new doctor. After office hours I made my introductory calls on the notables in town: the priest, the rabbi, the superintendent of the school. But the doorbell didn't ring the third day, or on the fourth or fifth day either. I drove up into the hills, where snow had already settled on the tall fir trees. At night I ate dinner alone at the inn and walked home through pitch-dark streets without meeting a living soul. I telephoned Maria.

Exactly one week after I had begun practicing, I was called to the house of my first patient. Her name was Sonnenschein, and she lived on a hill, in the last building of the ghetto. I can still see that little figure, with its birdlike face, sitting up in bed, wrapped in several blankets. She had a metastatic breast cancer, and I noted morphine ampoules on the bedside table. When I opened my bag and took out a syringe, she clutched the blankets to her. "Please, don't hurt me, *Herr Doktor*," she said.

I gave her the injection. She took a deep breath. "It did not hurt much," she said. "No more than when Dr. Klinger gave me the needle."

"Why should it hurt you more?" I said.

"Because people say that you're new."

I thought, Now at least the Jewish community will know that I don't murder people.

My second patient came from the gentile community, soon after Frau Sonnenschein called me. It was on a Sunday morning that my doorbell rang for the first time. I looked out the window and saw a young hunter helping an older one down from a peasant cart. The older man was pale and perspiring, his left arm in a sling; blood trickled through a dressing that had been clumsily applied. In my treatment room he collapsed, and we carried him to the couch. His escort gave the history.

The patient was the chief gamekeeper of the Duke's estate, and he had been injured when a gentleman hunter's rifle went off accidentally. I cut open the dressing, discovered the source of bleeding—a minor artery—quickly ligated it, and closed the wound with a few stitches. Then I removed some grains of shot that had lodged under the skin.

Meanwhile, the patient recovered and asked for water. "Wine would be better," he said, smacking his lips. His face regained its natural complexion—freckled from forehead to chin. With his healthy hand he brushed his close-cropped flaming red hair, then put on his hunter's cap, which was adorned with a long feather. "My name is Ferdl," he said and shook my hand. "I was Dr. Klinger's patient all my life, and I'm happy to meet his successor. I have confidence in Jewish doctors."

He must have spoken kindly about the new doctor's ability, because the following day two patients arrived from Neustift an der Rosalia, the village in which Ferdl lived, and one week later, when he arrived to have the stitches removed, I had treated a dozen patients.

I told him that his wound had healed fast.

"Hounds' bones heal fast," he said, quoting an old proverb. He smiled broadly, showing healthy teeth, with one front tooth missing. He told me he had lost it on the Italian front, where in a hand-to-hand fight it was knocked out by an enemy's gun barrel. He asked me whether I was interested in rifle practice, and when I said yes he invited me to the castle court, where there was a rifle range.

A few days later I drove up to Burg Forchtenstein. Snow had fallen the previous night, but the courtyard was brushed clean. Ferdl received me with a broad smile. The view from the watchtower into the valley was superb. We practiced target-shooting for more than an hour. I was a good shot, but Ferdl was, of course, much better. He enjoyed himself tremendously when he hit a bull's-eye. Finally we gave our rifles to the helper, and Ferdl invited me to the wine cellar. There we sat down at a rough, unpolished table, and Ferdl filled the glasses.

"Prosit," he said. "To many happy shootings. You *are* good!"

My practice increased. There was no lack of work that winter, for it was a bad season for flu and pneumonia. My first patient, poor old Frau Sonnenschein, died in late January.

All this, of course, I reported to Maria in nightly calls. Sometimes she was not home, and I would worry about my defeated rival, Ernst. Or had a new rival appeared?

"No," Maria said. "And what about you? A beautiful village maiden is making eyes at my Turkish potentate?"

"This is not a village," I said. "It is a *town*." I did not report that payments were few and far between. In Mattersburg there seemed to be an odd reluctance to pay for the doctor's services.

Around the beginning of February, Ferdl needed my attention again. A young hunter summoned me at five in the morning. He tried to dissuade me from using my car, and when I still insisted, he shrugged. "You'll see," he said.

It had rained during the night, and the road was flooded in several places. Still, I managed to navigate my Opel-Steyr up the winding route that led to the castle. Here the main road ended. Ferdl's house was a few kilometers beyond, but I didn't dare continue along the narrow, rutted path. While I deliberated, I heard the labored grinding of a horse and cart, which emerged bearing the tall figure of Ferdl topped by his hunter's hat.

On the way to his house, Ferdl told me that his wife had expectorated blood while lighting a fire on the kitchen hearth. She hadn't been feeling well since early the previous summer, coughed a great deal, and was losing weight. I listened and asked one or two questions. The symptoms, unless there were additional ones, easily suggested tuberculosis.

The car stopped at a neat house with a tiled roof, surrounded by chestnut trees, on which still hung a few thorny chestnut shells emptied of their contents. The air was crisp. I felt grateful for the sudden warmth of the kitchen. Two girls, about twelve and thirteen, and an older girl of about twenty waited for us.

In the adjoining room the patient lay under voluminous quilts. Her face was waxen, and her large eyes, so typical of tubercular patients, looked at me inquisitively. The examination proved that she was an advanced case.

Back in the kitchen, the family gathered around me. The two younger girls clearly resembled their parents, taking their blond hair and narrow, fragile faces from their mother, and the freckles and curved noses from their father. The eldest girl, a beautiful creature, buxom, with brown eyes, was the maid.

Tears ran down Ferdl's cheeks when I gave my prognosis. "Are you sure, *Herr Doktor?*" he said, wiping the tears from the corners of his eyes with his fist.

I replied that I was, but would confirm it by X ray if his wife could be brought to my office. When, I asked, had she started coughing?

Ferdl thought for a while. "It was around the strawberry harvest—the end of June, about."

"Did you take her to the doctor?"

"Yes, to Dr. Klinger, about the same time."

"And what did he say?"

"He examined her and said she had bronchitis. He gave her a prescription."

"And you never took her back?"

"Dr. Klinger said it would get better, and I often renewed the prescription."

The following day a chest X ray of Ferdl's wife showed both lungs riddled with cavities. Ferdl—as expected—refused hospitalization for his wife, which I suggested to protect the young people from contagion. What was required, then, was only care. The young maid volunteered to look after the patient. She was the granddaughter of the local midwife, and she had been taught how to nurse, she said.

For the first time I took a day off, which of course I spent with Maria. I told her how richly satisfying life in the country had proved to be. "You are too thin," she said. We were at the Kursalon, and she ordered a hot chocolate with whipped cream for me.

When I got back to my office, a cart was standing at the door. It belonged to a peasant, who told me that he had been waiting for several hours for my return. His little girl was sick, and his wife had instructed him that she wanted no other doctor. As soon as we set out, it started snowing again, and it took an hour to reach the top of the hill where he lived. The child had diphtheria. After treating her, I climbed back into the cart. The storm had developed into a blizzard, and the strong peasant horse struggled its way down the roads. By the time I arrived back in town, grayish daylight was filtering through thick clouds. Vienna had faded in my memory.

When Ferdl's wife died, in March, he retired from society, declining to drink wine with his neighbors, politely rejecting an invitation to visit me, and shunning the weekly target-shooting in the courtyard. People saw him walking aimlessly in the woods, accompanied by his two beagles, which, with drooping ears, seemed to participate in their master's grief.

I was pleasantly surprised one day a month later to discover him among my patients in the waiting-room. When his turn came, he insisted upon waiting until last. I was puzzled.

He entered my office, nervously fumbling with his cap, and peered back into the waiting-room before I closed the door. "Are you sure, *Herr Doktor,* that no one can overhear?" he said anxiously.

I reassured him.

He took a deep breath, then wiped his brow with a large handkerchief. "She seemed such a good girl," he said.

"Who?"

"Resl, our maid."

"What's wrong?"

Ferdl sighed. "She's expecting a baby, and she claims it's

mine." He slumped into a chair and buried his head in his large hands.

I tried hard not to laugh at this classic gesture of despair. The young girl had made a favorable impression on me. She had been good to the dying woman and seemed to be on the best of terms with the two daughters. "Come, now," I said, patting him on the back. "Congratulations are in order."

"No," he said. "It's not mine." He stood up and began to pace the room. "Her father and I were on the Italian front. He died. When I came home after the war, I heard that his wife had also died, of Spanish influenza, and their girl—she was then about eight—had been taken by her grandmother. Have you ever met Frau Handler, her grandmother? Well, you will one day. She must be close to ninety, but she still attends to her work as a midwife. Once the town council thought it was time to replace her with a younger woman. They found one who had just graduated from the midwife school in Vienna. She took the job, but she wasn't lucky. The first two children she delivered died during birth. People said that while the women were in labor they saw Resl's grandmother hobbling around their houses, and some claim they even saw her riding on a broom. I don't believe such nonsense, do you? Well, at any rate, the young midwife was fired, and the old woman took over again. People wanted to play safe. Then last summer, when my wife became too weak to do the household chores and tend the garden, we looked for a maid. Frau Handler came with her granddaughter. She said life was hard, and she kept talking about my friendship with her dead son. You know how old women carry on."

I nodded.

"I never liked that woman," he said. "She has been a gossip all her life, cutting people to pieces. But that day she talked and talked, and finally I gave in. And now I am the victim."

"But if you are not the father, why worry?"

"Because already everybody has heard the news. Even the Most

Reverend *Herr Pfarrer* congratulated me this morning when I was in the church."

"Look, Ferdl," I said, "I'm a doctor. I treat illnesses, patients. What can I do about gossip?"

"First, let me tell you what happened," he said. "After my wife died, I sent Resl home to her grandmother. I thought that my two daughters could keep house themselves. The girl left, apparently in good spirits. And then a few days later, when I came home one afternoon, I found the old midwife sitting at the kitchen table. As soon as I entered, she got up and hobbled over to me. 'Congratulations, Ferdl,' she said. She all but embraced me. 'Resl is pregnant." I told her I knew it. I didn't pay much attention. Pregnancy out of wedlock is nothing new among these country girls. I still didn't know what she wanted from me. Wasn't Resl pregnant when she left my house? she asked. I said, was I the only man in the world? And so one word led to another, and finally I told her to get out. Later I was sorry; after all, she was an old woman. But she really made me angry."

"Then?"

"I didn't hear anything more until a few days ago. Suddenly people began to hint at things, and finally the gossip was right out in the open. She did a good job, that witch." Ferdl sank into a chair. I worried about the cap with the long feather, which he was twisting in his hands.

"Believe me," I said, "you have the sympathy of another man. But I don't know what I can do."

"You can do everything, *Herr Doktor*. I remember a case of a pregnant girl in town. She and her mother accused a man, and he denied it. The man went to Dr. Klinger. He called the two scoundrels to his office. And after they came out they said they had lied. Dr. Klinger was a great man. He helped everybody. Talk to Frau Handler."

Three days later I spotted Frau Handler in my waiting room.

It was not hard to recognize her. When she sat down in the chair facing me I found a striking resemblance between her eyes and the brown eyes of her granddaughter. The eyes alone retained a spark of youth.

"Do you know who I am?" she asked.

I said that I did.

"Then you probably know the reason for my coming."

"Well," I said evasively, "you're the midwife, aren't you?"

She nodded. "Do you know Ferdl, the gamekeeper?"

"He is my patient," I said.

"Well then, you can be of great help. Ferdl is shirking his duties as the father of a newborn child."

"It was born?" I asked in surprise.

"This morning at four. A little boy—four kilograms—with fire-red hair and a lot of it. Even freckles!"

"Congratulations."

"*Danke schön.*" The old woman played nervously with the wings of her kerchief. "*Herr Doktor,* I came here to ask you to persuade the villain of his duty."

"But Ferdl denies it flatly," I said.

"Aha!" She laughed. "A fine gentleman! First he leads a good, innocent girl astray, then he says, 'Not me—somebody else.' "

"And what does Resl say?"

"Resl says nothing. You can talk and plead and shout, and that stupid goose simply cries."

"Then how can you prove it?"

"How? Very simple. Look at the baby. The image of his father —the hair and the big hands. Listen, do you know who delivered Ferdl himself? I did, and I remember every child I ever delivered. I remember Ferdl—the hair and the hands. When I saw those hands, I said that he would become a hunter one day, and a good one."

Next morning I went up to the midwife's house. Like Ferdl's, it was in the forest, but nearer to the castle. It was a cottage with a tiny garden around it; smoke wafted from the chimney. Twenty-four hours after delivery, Resl was already on her feet, and when I entered the house she was bathing the baby happily. When I looked at the baby, I was thunderstruck. It *was* the image of Ferdl.

Resl lifted up the homely creature. "Isn't it wonderful?" she said.

The old woman was hobbling around, pouring water into a large pail on the hearth. She turned to Resl. "Now speak up," she said.

At once Resl began to cry.

"Stupid goose," Frau Handler said. "You see, she is hopeless. What can be done? She cannot live in shame and raise a child without a father. You must speak with that *Bösewicht, Herr Doktor.*"

I threw up my hands. "I'll see what I can do."

"*Bitte,*" she said, and as I left she muttered, "Why is old Dr. Klinger not here?"

I drove up to Ferdl's house. He was cleaning his rifle while the beagles stood and watched with boredom. He expressed surprise at seeing me at such an early hour. I usually made house calls late in the afternoon.

"I just visited Resl," I said. "She has a baby, a little boy."

"So?" he said, without interrupting his work.

"The baby has red hair and large hands."

He looked up. "And so?"

"It speaks for itself," I said.

"Am I the only man with red hair and big hands?" He laughed. "You'd better have a glass of wine, *Herr Doktor.* I think the old woman has bewitched you."

The arrival of the little red-haired boy was the topic of conversation everywhere I went. Women in black kerchiefs leaned out of their windows to question me; men stopped me on the street.

Public opinion was convinced of the hunter's paternity, and so was I.

My leave of absence was nearing its end, and I decided to resume my residency in Vienna. I knew that I must catch up with things I had missed since leaving the hospital. Also I missed Maria, despite our phone conversations, and I worried about rivals, who are always more dangerous and handsome when seen in the imagination.

Practice slowed down a bit after the winter months, and I enrolled in a postgraduate course in hematology, which had developed into a pillar of modern medicine. The research work of Dr. Landsteiner, a Viennese doctor who in 1930 received the Nobel Prize for discovering the so-called blood groups, had begun thirty years earlier, and we had already learned in medical school about these four blood groups: A, B, AB, and O. The large majority of Western people belonged to group O, and the rest were divided between A and B. Only five per cent belonged to group AB.

It was an unusually hot day in April when I attended the first session of the course. After the lecturer had given some basic information about recent advances in hematology, he turned to complicated theoretical interpretations. The room was steaming, and the numbers and letters on the blackboard seemed to fuse. But then suddenly I heard something of which I recall, even now, almost every word.

"There is a by-product of the research in the blood-group field —although it belongs more in the province of legal medicine," said the lecturer, Dr. Halter, a thin, slightly bent middle-aged man, with a spry mustache. "Paternity can be *disproved* if the child and the accused father do not belong to the same blood grouping."

I could hardly wait until the lecture finished. I followed Dr. Halter into his laboratory and told him about Ferdl, Resl, and the midwife.

"*Aber, Herr Kollege,*" he said after I concluded my story, "everything is still part of a research program. It would never stand a chance in court—and I wouldn't be part of it."

"It wouldn't go to court. Word of honor."

"Don't look for trouble," he said.

I kept on talking, and finally Dr. Halter took a deep breath. "All right," he said. "Bring samples of the blood of the child and of that hunter, although I doubt that he will submit."

The following morning, at six, I was at the midwife's house.

"Well," she said, "has he owned up to it?"

"No," I said, "but we'll try something else." We settled down at the kitchen table, and I proceeded as simply as possible to explain the theory of the blood groups to her. Those young brown eyes were fixed on me. "Now, you see," I said, "if the baby belongs to one of those groups, and Ferdl to another, then it is not his baby."

"And whose is it?" she asked defiantly.

"Let me finish. Even if they should have the same group— Well, it is not positive evidence, I must warn you." I cleared my throat and began a theoretical explanation. The more I progressed, the more I became confused. I was ready to give up when the old woman interrupted me.

"Look, *Herr Doktor,*" she said, "I've been a midwife for sixty-five years. When we started, we didn't wash our hands with soap and chlor water before we helped to deliver. Many, many mothers died of fever. But then we heard of that doctor—Semmelweis—and we were told to wash our hands. I didn't understand, but I did it. I don't understand what those blood groups mean, but I believe in science."

She assisted me, and I drew 5 c.c.s from the baby's arm.

I went on to Ferdl's house.

Ferdl listened to my explanation without interruption. After I finished, he shook his head as though dazed. "I can hit a hare from three hundred meters, and the bull's-eye ten times in a row, as you know, but I don't understand one single word you have said. But you must know what you are talking about. Go ahead."

I packed the two vials into my bag and set out for Vienna.

Dr. Halter typed the baby's blood first. It belonged to the rarest group—AB. I held my breath when Dr. Halter typed Ferdl's blood. It too was AB. I felt jubilant.

Dr. Halter bit his mustache. "It's still only a probability, remember," he warned me.

I made the trip home in half an hour less than usual and drove straight to Ferdl. "The baby and you belong to the same blood group," I said sternly.

Ferdl glanced around, and his eyes met mine. He shrugged. "Well," he said. "Science must know best."

That evening a strange procession came to my office: a dozen Jewish firemen in uniform. Although the Jewish community was an integral part of the town, the fire department of the Jews had retained its medieval status of autonomy. This fire department had a great reputation among Jews and gentiles alike. If fire broke out even in a remote village, the Jewish firemen could be counted on to arrive first. The firemen informed me that in a special meeting I had been elected president of the fire department. I answered that I felt honored, but my knowledge of fire-fighting was negligible. They assured me that no special knowledge on my part was required. I consented, thinking that my position would be purely honorary.

A fortnight later I was wakened by voices in the street. When I looked out the window, I saw my firemen standing around their engine.

"Hurry up, *Herr Doktor!*" they shouted. "There's a fire in Antau!" A minute later a helmet was being squeezed over my head and I was being helped into a fireman's blouse. The boots I pulled up while I was sitting in the engine.

The Jewish firemen got to Antau first.

Since my leave of absence from the hospital was soon to expire, I went to Vienna to request from my chief another half-year of leave. I finished my speech to him with the words: "Can I abandon my fire department?"

Later I said the same thing to Maria. "What did your chief say?" she asked.

"He said, 'I suppose not.' "

"So I suppose I must say the same. Do you have much of this fire-department work?"

"Very little."

"Good," she said. "You are still too thin, badly in need of *gute Hausmannskost.*"

DIAGNOSING THE RABBI

The additional half-year was up. We had not "rushed into marriage"; Maria and marriage and even the hospital apartment, now available, were waiting for me in Vienna. It was no use; I could not leave Mattersburg.

I went to Vienna and tried to explain my feelings to Maria. When I finished, I thought the twelve-year-old girl had returned; that was how her face looked. In a moment she would stick out her tongue at me.

"All right," she said. "Then I'll come to Mattersburg."

Our wedding, on April 27, 1930, was only the final act in a series of exciting events connected with establishing a household. Pieces of furniture we had bought in Vienna refused to enter the Mattersburg apartment. I suggested sawing off a bit here and another there, offered to do it myself, and was asked if I had gone out of my mind. Other pieces had no difficulty getting in but, once in, immediately quarreled with their surroundings, or so Maria said. All these pieces had to be exchanged. It seems to me now, as I look back, that the only items we had no trouble with were the pots and pans. And all the time, all around me—as I argued and expostulated and rushed to Vienna to ponder with Maria over the color of a living-room rug and rushed back again —there was the winter's harvest of pneumonia, plus heart cases and bronchitis and diphtheria and measles and the common, common cold.

We were married at the Seitenstetten Tempel, which was noted for especially formal weddings, but Maria refused to wear white and would have nothing to do with a veil in any circumstances. She appeared in a dress of sea-foam green and of course looked stunning. Everything went well. I squeezed her hand during the ceremony, and she squeezed back. Since I had rehearsed the delicate wedding-ring maneuver again and again, I anticipated no trouble; the ring waited securely in my lower left vest pocket. I was asked for it and confidently put my finger in the pocket to draw it out. Of course it was not there. Nor was it in the right-hand lower vest pocket, nor in any other. This was such a familiar situation in books and plays and films that I did not believe it was happening.

"There it is," Maria whispered. The ring was on the little finger of my left hand.

After the ceremony she asked why I had put it there.

"I didn't," I said.

"Then who did?" she asked. The question was unanswerable and remains a mystery to this day.

We were to spend the honeymoon, for which my practice would allow only one week, on the Semmering, a mountain resort with two big hotels that were famous for honeymoons; but Maria selected instead a small, charming inn that had once upon a time been a tiny rococo-baroque castle. The ceiling of our room reached to heaven, and it was bitter cold; even the huge blazing fire hardly helped, unless you stood close enough to roast yourself. We had *Himmelbetten* (fourposters) just like those to be seen at Schönbrunn, where Maria Theresa and her spouse had slept.

On the second evening I was called to the telephone. From Mattersburg, Herr Spiegel, whose wife I had delivered a week ago, reported in a quaking voice that she was feverish.

We took the night train.

Frau Spiegel recovered in a few days, but who can resume an interrupted honeymoon?

Maria had taken a cooking course with all the trimmings and graduated with honors, but our first meal at home seemed resolved to follow the great comic tradition of newlyweds' first meals, just as I had followed another tradition with the wedding ring. Pea soup, veal goulash with Nockerln and poppy-seed noodles. How can pea soup turn brown? How can it *not* taste of peas? The veal had spent a long life thundering up and down the Argentine pampas before dying of exhaustion and the despondency of the aged. The noodles were more like a strudel. With shining eyes Maria watched me eat. She herself was too excited to take even one bite. "Good?" she asked.

"Sublime," I said as I strongly chewed. "How did you do it?"

"It is all a matter of careful preparation," she replied. What a wonderful cook she was to become!

The next day Frau Klinger came to call. I introduced her to Maria. As they smiled and murmured polite words, young doctor's wife, old doctor's widow, perhaps one was thinking: Will I be like her one day?—and the other, Once upon a time I was like her. The old lady had brought a large bundle. She unwrapped it and revealed pots and pans, two framed prints (the first, Mattersburg besieged by the Turks; the second, a young man with pointed mustache), and a book. Frau Klinger pointed to the young man, then touched her eyes with a lace handkerchief. "My poor husband," she said. "I thought you would like to have it to hang in your consulting room, also the other print. The pots and pans are for you, my dear," she added to Maria. She said nothing about the book.

Maria prepared coffee and cake—rather like clay—and I ex-
cused myself to make house calls. "Just like my husband," the old
lady said, "always on the run. I must leave myself in a few minutes."

Four hours later, when I returned, she was still sitting there
giving advice to Maria. I went to my office, saw two patients, did
some paperwork, and returned to the living room. "Another
thing you must always remember," Frau Klinger was saying," is
to—" She saw me. "Ah, *Herr Doktor,* I have been waiting for
you." She picked up the book. "This is my poor husband's medical library. I am giving it to you." And with a solemn gesture she
put it into my hand. "He read it again and again. People will tell
you he did not read it in vain. Now I must really be off."

The book's worn old cover still showed a design of stylized field
flowers.

DR. ZIFFER KÁROLY
ORVOSI TANACSADO

This edition, the twelfth, of Dr. Charles Ziffer's medical text-
book had been printed in Budapest in 1876, and so it must have
been written in the 1860s or even 1850s. I turned the pages. In the
margin here and there Dr. Klinger's fine handwriting appeared.
On the sixth page he had drawn attention with big letters to the
importance of the subject: Hyperhydrosis (perspiration of the
feet). I read that sudden disappearance of foot perspiration might
have tremendous consequences for the general health and there-
fore the treatment to eliminate it must be applied with the utmost
care. The very best method was a tepid foot-bath (not hot and
not cold!). I glanced through the next couple of hundred pages
and came to diseases of lesser importance: Diseases of the heart.
Treatment: no coffee; no alcohol; careful regulation of the bowel
movement; no irritation. Above all, the patient must avoid physical exertion.

The book brought back childhood memories: Dr. Klinger's

house, window sills filled with pots of geraniums; patients lined up all day in the courtyard under the walnut trees—he did not believe in waiting-rooms. Sometimes I dared to peek into his mysterious office with its pungent smell of alcohol and iodine and dust. There were two chairs, an old table that served as a desk, and a rickety examining table. In one corner a tall cabinet held the doctor's instruments. I had thought there were a lot of them but, looking back, I realized there could not have been more than half a dozen, if that.

Dr. Klinger was a short man with a comfortable paunch and a face that seldom smiled. I was always glad when he invited me to ride around with him on his house calls. In the winter he looked really impressive because he owned a mighty fur coat, and when you saw him sitting with calm, unsmiling face in the back seat of his carriage you could not help thinking that he must be a very great doctor indeed. It was difficult territory that we covered in that carriage, especially in winter—from valley to mountaintop, one patient's house many kilometers from the next. Still, Dr. Klinger said, he would not change his practice for that of a *Nichts-tuer* doctor in Vienna. As the carriage slowly climbed the serpentine road to Burg Forchtenstein he told me about the brave imperial soldiers who had defended it against the Turks. He spoke so proudly that he might have been one of them.

I turned the pages. Here was a list of medications. Digitalis wasn't mentioned. Could there really have been a time when digitalis wasn't used in treating heart disease?

"People will tell you he did not read it in vain," the old lady had said. And at the door she had added, "Read it too, *Herr Doktor!* Read it well!"

Frau Sonnenschein was the only Jewish patient I had had, and I wondered why.

Then one day I had a visit from a boy with a wide-brimmed hat and curls in front of his ears, who summoned me to the house

of Rabbi Sobelstein. This was not the almighty Chief Rabbi but
his deputy, the nominal dean of the local Talmudic school, which
had a great reputation among Orthodox Jews far and wide. The
boy in the wide-brimmed hat was a student. When I asked him if
it was Rabbi Sobelstein who was ill or a member of his family, he
shrugged.

He led me down Jew Street to a building across from the fif-
teenth-century synagogue. The door was baroque, the building
itself plain Renaissance, with a narrow courtyard, loggias, brittle
walls that had probably not been painted for centuries. We went
up a winding staircase, through a small foyer, and into a large
room with whitewashed walls, a huge table, and two chairs. In
one of them sat Rabbi Sobelstein.

Gently his body moved from side to side as he read from a big
book with parchment pages. Apparently he hadn't noticed us,
and I did not want to disturb him. The boy quietly left. Finally
the rabbi looked up. He saw me and smiled through his great
gray beard. Of course my bag told him who I was.

"Have you been here long, *Herr Doktor?* You should have said
something. Doctors have better things to do than watch an old
man." He stood up and immediately began to undress—first the
caftan, then a shirt, then another, and then an undershirt, and so
on until he was naked.

I was puzzled. "What is wrong with you, Rabbi?" I asked.

"Are you not the doctor?" he said gently.

He was a tall, very thin man; his ribs stood out, but otherwise
he looked healthy. I listened to his heart and his lungs and took
his blood pressure. "Don't trouble to examine the abdomen," he
told me. "My digestion is perfect." There was no hernia; his reflexes were normal.

Well, I was ready to give an opinion. "There's nothing wrong
with you, Rabbi."

"Nothing?"

I looked into the mellow eyes. I thought hard. He had flat feet. Could that be called a sickness?

"Any backache?" I said.

He began to dress. With deliberation he buttoned his suspenders and put on the caftan. He sat down and smiled. "You have made the correct diagnosis," he said.

"Then, Rabbi," I said, "you need arch supports in your shoes." I put away my stethoscope and blood-pressure machine.

"Can you spare a few minutes, *Herr Doktor?*"

"Yes, of course."

"Good. People come closer to each other when they talk. Tell me, how do you like it in our little town? You are accustomed to life in the big city, aren't you?"

"I don't have any real complaints, Rabbi."

"People are different in a little town, I would say a bit suspicious." He looked at me. "In short, *Herr Doktor,* they are used to a man like Dr. Klinger. Fifty years is a long time, *nicht wahr?* He grew old and became the way some old men are, impatient, a bit morose; but, all in all, *ein ganzer Mensch.* And a good diagnostician. When he gave his opinion it sounded like a judge's verdict."

His long thin fingers wandered through the beard's luxuriant tangle.

"I hope you won't mind if I ask you how old you are, *Herr Doktor.*"

"Twenty-nine, Rabbi."

"So young. My mother used to say a doctor was no good until he'd filled up a cemetery or two." He smiled again. "Yet I've heard that nowadays there are some young doctors who also know their business. Some peasants from the villages talk of you quite kindly. And now I can too, *Herr Doktor!*"

Once again I had the feeling of having passed an examination. "Thank you, Rabbi."

"One word more. I am happy that you married a good Jewish

girl, and that she buys kosher meat. And we hope you'll come to the synagogue, at least for the High Holidays. Will you?"

I told him I would do my best.

But if some peasants had spoken of me "quite kindly," it appears that others had not. "There are complaints against you, *Herr Doktor,*" Ferdl said. "They liked the way they were treated by Dr. Klinger. He never talked much, and he didn't have to look at you very much either—sometimes not at all. I remember when my little girl got sick around midnight and I hurried to town and rang the doctor's bell. The *Frau Doktor* looked out the window. 'What's wrong, Ferdl?' she asked. 'Mitzi can't swallow and she's hot all over,' I said. 'Wait,' she said and pulled her head in. After a while she stuck it out again. 'Here,' she said and threw down a piece of paper. It was the doctor's prescription. I woke up the pharmacist, he made it up, I took the medicine home, and the next day Mitzi was all right."

We were having a glass of wine after target-shooting. Ferdl refilled my glass. "The trouble with you, *Herr Doktor,* you spend too much time with your patients. And often you put them behind the Roentgen machine."

"The Roentgen machine represents modern medicine."

"It makes them uneasy. Dr. Klinger would never use it."

That was true. Dr. Klinger had applied splints and plaster casts without benefit of X-ray diagnosis. Once, I remember, I remarked about it. "Do you see more crippled people here than in Vienna?" he asked sharply.

Despite criticism, I was not going to give up the Roentgen machine. One day even the most stupid peasant would learn to overcome his uneasy feeling and thank the machine for possibly having saved his life.

The news of my brilliant diagnosis of Rabbi Sobelstein's flat feet spread like wildfire through the ghetto, and one night the Chief Rabbi himself summoned me.

His residence was above the rabbinical school. There was the usual winding staircase, but the rooms had an atmosphere of *noblesse*. The Chief Rabbi of Mattersburg (the historical name was Mattersdorf) was known far beyond the borders of Austria. Even now, when the ghetto and its famous rabbinical school are only a memory, if I mention to a Jewish patient that I once practiced there I can see the awe in his face. It was an honor to study under the great rabbi, and students came from all over Europe and even from America.

What an aristocratic figure he was, the *Herr Oberrabbiner!* A tall, strongly built man, he had a pitch-black beard that shone, and his almond-shaped eyes under long lashes looked candidly and earnestly at you, as they did at me this night when he told me about a feverish child. His daughter had chicken pox, I found. It wouldn't make sense to isolate the other children, I told him and his anxious wife, because the incubation period had already started. All would be well.

From then on I was a steady guest in the rabbi's house. Often, as we talked, I would hear the singsong voices of the students in the school below.

There had been seven historical Jewish communities in the Burgenland; the Mattersburg *Oberrabbiner* was the spiritual chief of all. He came from a long line of rabbis. I remember the first time he took me to his study, an octagonal room with a high ceiling and tiny grated windows. Originally it must have been the watchtower of a medieval building, which had gone through several architectural periods until it reached the baroque, where it had stayed.

"Wie geht es Ihnen, Herr Doktor?" he asked with a smile, and as I write the words I can smell the old books and folios. There on his desk was the latest issue of the *Neue Freie Presse;* the rabbi was interested in worldly affairs. I cannot remember a single instance of his attempting to proselytize me; indeed, he forgave my many infractions. Once he was asked why he continued to regard

me as a friend while he was uncompromising with the slightest deviations from Orthodox ritual on the part of members of his flock. "Our doctor is a *gehaimer Zaddik*," he explained. This was the first time I had heard myself described as a "secretly devout" man.

On the other hand, I never did anything to offend the Jewish community. I never drove through the *Judengasse* on the Sabbath, and, as Rabbi Sobelstein had noted, Maria always bought kosher meat. On the Day of Atonement and the other official days of mourning (God knows Jews have had reason to mourn during their long history) only the ill were exempted from ritual requirements, and the doctor had to certify that they *were* ill. "When you certify," the rabbi said with a twinkle when I told him that Herr Klein or Frau Kohn was in no position to fast, "kindly use my standards."

There was a half-dimness, one might say the shadow of a shadow, in his study even during daylight hours, and sometimes it seemed to throw a shadow across the almond eyes. He did not like the look of the future, he said. "But *Shemisborach* (may His Name be forever blessed) will help us once again, as He helped us so often when we were on the very brink. Mighty empires have disappeared. We are still here." And he got up and, as he was in the habit of doing, walked to one of the narrow windows and looked down on the small creek, the Wulka, peaceful and shining in the sun.

Many years later I went to a housing project on the Lower East Side to visit an old friend and talk about our vanished world. He opened the door and smiled through the great beard, now snow-white. In this modern apartment there was the same atmosphere of *noblesse,* and the same aroma of old books. "Your son," the rabbi said, "a big doctor now, isn't he? Do you remember when you brought him to see me the first time? He couldn't have been more than two and a half. And what did he do? He sang a song."

How well I remembered that song, and little Peter singing it out full blast in the Chief Rabbi's face! It was a song I used to sing driving around on house calls, with Peter beside me:

> *Wenn die Soldaten durch die Stadt marschieren*
> *Öffnen die Mädchen die Fenster und die Türen!*
> When the soldiers march in the streets
> The girls open their doors and windows!

"Time passes," the rabbi said. And he got up and walked to the window and looked down on the East River, as he used to look down on small Wulka creek.

During the summer my practice fell off, and Maria and I drove up into the hills, she in a dirndl, I in leather shorts and Tyrolean *Janker*. They were the best months of our lives; we were in full harmony except that I liked to sing an aria after reaching the mountaintop. Love and happiness had enormously improved my voice, I was convinced, but Maria declared the contrary to be the case; marriage, she said, had ruined it. Anyway, she didn't like opera—which remains true to this day.

Beginning almost with the first days of fall, my waiting-room was crammed, and I also made many house calls. Returning from one, I found Maria with a somber face. "It cannot go on like this," she said. "Do you realize that we don't have a single groschen in the house?"

"Impossible," I said.

"Impossible? *Impossible?* I've been through every drawer! The kitchen light went dead; we don't have any spare bulbs, and there's no money to buy one. Something has to be done, Richard."

"All right," I said.

"Your bills are never paid. You are going to send out reminders, starting *now*."

But I had no reminder forms with my letterhead. I thougﬁt I'd have to get them from Vienna, then learned that there was a printing shop in the town in the *Judengasse.*

I went to Jew Street, looking for the printer's sign, but couldn't find it. Then I heard a rattling sound. I crossed a courtyard formed by walls with protruding Renaissance loggias. The room I entered was dimly lit by a kerosene lamp hanging over the rattling press. The printer couldn't have heard me come in. He was small, somewhat bent. I tapped him on the shoulder, and he gave a little start as he turned. So did I. He wore an old spiked helmet. A Jewish printer in spiked helmet is an unusual sight.

I shouted my name. He stopped the press and looked at me with respect. "Sorry not to have met you before, *Herr Doktor.* It's my fault; I'm never sick." He grinned at his joke.

"Can you print some reminders for me?" I asked.

"Reminders?" he said.

"You are a printer, aren't you?"

"Of course. But—"

As I looked at his frowning face, I couldn't help smiling, not because of the spiked helmet but because of an old story I suddenly remembered. A man's wristwatch stops; he looks for a watchmaker, sees a window filled with watches, goes into the shop, finds an old Jew with mighty beard behind the counter. "Can you repair this?" he says, taking off the watch. "Repair it? I'm not a watchmaker," says the old man. "Then what are you?" "I'm a *moil* [one who performs circumcisions]." "Then what are those watches doing in your window?" "You'll tell me, maybe, what else I should put there?"

The printer looked reproachfully at me, as though saying "It's so funny, what I said?"

"They're called reminders because they're supposed to remind the patient of the bill he hasn't paid," I explained. "It's an exception if one of my patients pays."

The printer reached into the pocket of his apron, and squeezed out some tobacco followed by a cigarette paper. He rolled the cigarette, lit it, deeply inhaled, exhaled, and watched the curling smoke. "Please listen, *Herr Doktor*," he said. "Our old town has gone through a lot in its history. The Tartars came in the thirteenth century and burned it to the ground. It was rebuilt. Then the Turks came. They were more decent; after they found they couldn't conquer Burg Forchtenstein they went away without burning the town, only taking the young boys with them. I could tell you many more interesting events, *Herr Doktor,* but there is one thing our old town has never seen: a doctor who sends out reminders."

"But why not?" I asked.

"We are an agricultural community with a few hundred stonemasons who go to Vienna to work; also we have our ancient ghetto with its storekeepers and artisans. The peasants, the fruitgrowers who live all around our town, have no cash; they have to wait for the harvest. The stonemasons don't work during the winter months because no one builds then. Our Jewish merchants depend on the money they get from the rest of the population. In one word, *Herr Doktor,* it's a vicious circle."

"It's certainly vicious for my wife and me," I said.

"*Geduld,*" he said. "But even if there were money around, *Herr Doktor,* would it be wise to send out reminders? Wouldn't it make people think, 'Aha! Our young doctor is poor!'? And between you and me, who likes or respects a poor man?"

"Well," I admitted, "I see your point, Herr—"

"Call me Aaron, everyone does."

"I see your point, Aaron, and I suppose I must just stick it out. Where did you learn so much about history, psychology, shrewd judgment?"

He crushed out the cigarette. "We printers," he said proudly, "are an elite."

On New Year's Day around five in the morning my doorbell rang, then rang again, and again. I looked out the window and saw, in the light of the street lamp (the only one in town) a man with a red beard. It was Schwarz the Seltzer (every merchant had a nickname). *"Herr Doktor,* hurry!" he shouted. "My wife is in labor, she's bleeding, and Frau Handler says she's going to die!"

A few minutes later Schwarz the Seltzer and I were running toward the *Judengasse.* Frau Handler, the old midwife, received me with gloomy face. "The baby doesn't move down, only blood comes out." She shrugged. *"Sie muss halt sterben."*

I quickly scrubbed, then examined Schwarz's wife. It was a case of *placenta previa:* the placenta blocked the uterus exit. The placenta's blood vessels had been ruptured by the contractions and stretchings. The baby was in a pelvic presentation—buttocks down. I was grateful for the training I had had at the Brigitta Spital, an auxiliary of the Vienna City Hospital. I made a hole through the placenta and pulled one leg through. The buttock acted as a tampon; the bleeding stopped instantly. (This method has been abandoned except in emergencies; Caesarian section is now used.)

The midwife's thousand deep wrinkles spread outward and made her old face bigger as she smiled. *"Na so was!"* she said. With a quick maneuver I extricated the baby. Frau Schwarz's face slowly regained its color. I washed my hands and was ready to leave.

"Herr Doktor," Schwarz the Seltzer said, "how can I thank you?"

"A hundred schillings," I said. Even by Mattersburg standards this was a modest fee.

He shook my hand but, needless to say, did not produce any money.

The next night when I came home from a call, I saw by Maria's face that something dramatic had happened. "What is it?" I asked.

"Come and see."

As I climbed the stairs my right foot caught. I looked down and saw the lever of a seltzer bottle. "What is a seltzer bottle doing here?" I asked Maria, but she did not reply. She opened the door to the corridor connecting my office with the rest of the apart-ment. "There you are," she said. "So!"

The corridor was filled with seltzer bottles. They stood neatly arranged in rows, like soldiers. Their ranks extended to the kitchen floor and even to the dining room.

"This afternoon," Maria said, "Herr Schwarz arrived. He blessed your name for what happened. Then he went to his horse and cart and began to take out seltzer bottles. I couldn't stop him, not even when he passed the hundred mark. Finally he mopped his brow and said, 'Two hundred seltzer bottles at fifty groschen each make one hundred schillings. Tell the *Herr Dok-tor* that I don't like to owe money.' "

"I see," I said.

"Yes? Please tell me what we're going to do with them."

"We will have to start drinking a lot of seltzer."

The next day I saw Aaron the Helmet standing at his door, smoking a cigarette. I told him about Schwartz the Seltzer's pay-ment. "Be glad it wasn't twins," Aaron the Helmet said.

Spring arrived overnight. The barren twigs of the trees and shrubs bore tender buds and then the *Baumblüte*—lily-white blossoms as far as the eye could see, only the church towers rising above the lovely fragrant foam. Another month, another, and the cherry season was here, followed by that of the *Ananas*—the local name for giant, juicy strawberries. Peasant carts slowly waddled off to the Vienna markets; trains bound for the city no longer smelled of smoke and tobacco; the passengers breathed the perfume of cherries and a million strawberries. On Sunday mornings before going to church men in their best clothes and shiny boots and their wives in big skirts and black kerchiefs paid the debts that had accumulated during the long winter. They brought baskets of cherries and strawberries to the merchants and the artisans —and to the doctor.

Every corner of our apartment, all storage spaces, even parts of my office were filled with baskets of fruit. At first Maria threw up her hands; then she got to work, steadily phoning friends and relatives to come and help themselves. Needless to say we ate a great deal and became very particular about the quality of the cherries and strawberries we consumed, choosing the very best. This was only the beginning; the apple, pear, and plum harvests followed.

And finally came the vintage. A wine-grower stopped me and invited me into his house. *"Nur einen Schluck, Herr Doktor."* Another mouthful at his neighbor's . . . another, and another. I reached home sitting in a vacant happy state in a peasant cart, my little Opel-Steyr attached behind by a rope. The next morning I opened my eyes to find Maria looking at me. I expected to hear Mändl's voice: "I thought I said one drink?" Or Mother's: "You are a doctor now. You must behave like one."

"At least we've got the money for a light bulb," I said.

In private practice, death has a far more traumatic impact than in the hospital, where the doctor is part of an establishment and the responsibilities are divided—although things are by no means always so simple.

I was summoned to the only Hebrew delicatessen in town. I knew the owner, Jishe, a man around forty with a big ginger-colored beard, always in good spirits. The small store, bursting with food and spicy smells, was a favorite gathering place, where there were many discussions and lively exchanges. Standing behind his counter, cutting and slicing, ladling out pickles, Jishe would join in. He was a pious Jew, respected even by the rabbi, and a man with manifold interests. I often stopped for a chat and a bite of something good. He had never been to my office. He never complained.

There was a large crowd in front of the delicatessen. I made my way through and into the shop. Jishe was lying behind his counter. All the hushed talk stopped as I knelt and listened. No heartbeat: Jishe was dead. I got up and put the stethoscope away. There was his wife, pale and trembling, and his children. What was I to say? What could I say? (How often I was to face the same situation in the next forty years!) But the other people understood at once, and the store was filled with the somber sound of the holiest of all Jewish prayers: *Sh'ma Yisroel Adonai Elohenu Adonai Echod* ("Hear, O Israel, the Lord our God is one God.")

Now Jishe's pale wife said, "But *Herr Doktor,* he was alive just a few minutes ago. He was telling me a funny story about something our littlest one did, when he stumbled and fell. Couldn't you— Isn't there something— If maybe you pricked him with a needle?"

Back at the office, the waiting-room was full. I ate my dinner without appetite (the days of mysterious brown pea soup had long since disappeared). I went to bed at ten. I couldn't sleep. I had told Maria about the death; she had said, "Then there was nothing you could do." It must have been eleven or even twelve when I thought: But is that true? Is Jishe *really* dead?

Had I done everything to make sure? Of course I had. I had diagnosed death hundreds of times in the hospital. Jishe had had a heart attack.

I turned over in bed. Maria was asleep.

I got up and dressed very quietly and soon was on my way to the *Judengasse.* It was a peaceful night with full moonshine. The ancient street was empty. All the windows of the old buildings were dark, except one. Filtered through a curtain, faint light came from above the delicatessen. I walked up one flight and entered the room where, according to Jewish ritual, Jishe lay on a heap of straw, a burning candle behind his head. In one corner a rabbinical student sat sound asleep, a holy book on his lap.

Jishe had been dressed in his best suit. I unbuttoned the vest and placed the stethoscope on his heart. There was no beat.

···
⊰ *xiii* ⊱

_____

THE *JUDENGASSE*,

A LOST WORLD

Since I had had my training in obstetrics at the Brigitta Spital, Maria was to go there to be delivered. Her obstetrician, the chief resident, anticipated that the happy event would occur on or around August 15. She went to Vienna on August 8. A number of hours pass between the first pains and delivery in a *primipara*, or first birth, and so I would have plenty of time to drive to the hospital. Of course, as so often seems to happen with doctors, I did not have plenty of time, because I was out making calls and they couldn't reach me.

The phone was ringing as I entered the apartment. I rushed to it. "Yes? Dr. Berczeller here!" I shouted.

"Congratulations," the obstetrician's voice said laconically. "It's a boy."

I did not believe my ears. For the first time I understood why young new fathers look the way they do when they hear the news. It was August 11.

Eight days later Maria came home with Peter Hanns. Dozens of presents had arrived, and now there were more. Ferdl brought a barrel of wine and a two-barrel shotgun. "Men must learn to drink early," he said, "also to shoot. I hope he will learn to shoot before he knows how to talk." At the time this seemed to me one of the most delightfully humorous remarks ever uttered, and I laughed my head off.

With this new life, a new life began for us, revolving around the baby. How often I was awakened in the middle of the night to hear Maria inform me in an agitated voice, "He doesn't drink. Why?" If I did not respond promptly with a rational and convincing explanation, she would call me a *Rabenvater* (are ravens really cruel fathers?). Half asleep, I would carry the fully awake baby up and down, up and down. I learned for the first time why young new fathers always look sleepy.

Before long Maria was taking Peter out in a baby carriage half the size of Father's Daimler—a present from him and Mother. "Everybody says Peter is big for his age," Maria told me. Another time she rushed after me as I left the living room to go to my office. "The baby followed you with his eyes!" she cried. "And he isn't even two months old! You must admit, Richard, he is perfectly wonderful!"

"He doesn't deserve any credit," I said humorously. "It is all due to the parents."

"Ah, you! *Rabenvater!"*

Often I would see Aaron standing in front of his door, which had a baroque handle carved with a symbolized serpent, and I'd stop for a chat. "I'm not too busy," he would explain. "Mostly I print prayer books. Well, how many can you print? There's no new version of the Bible."

He had never married and lived his bachelor life in one room with a kitchen stove in the corner. Packed bookshelves lined the walls: Goethe, Schiller, Heine, Lessing, and so on, but also Marx, Engels, Lassalle, Lenin, Rosa Luxemburg. Herzl's *Old New Land* was in a prominent place.

As our friendship developed, we got into political discussions.

He knew I was a Social Democrat; for decades Father had been one of the party leaders. "How is it you find so many Jewish intellectuals among the Socialists?" he asked.

"Socialism means progress," I said, "justice and equality."

"What's wrong with Zionism? Isn't the shirt closer to the body than the jacket? Shouldn't we think of us first? Justice for Jews?"

"That means that only a tiny percentage of mankind would benefit."

He gestured with his left hand; in the right, there was the inevitable cigarette. "We Jews!" he exclaimed. "We are the do-gooders throughout history, from Jesus to Marx—embracing the whole world in our loving arms, while it kicks us in the ass. *'Alle Menschen werden Brüder.'* " And he hummed the familiar bars from the Ninth Symphony.

"It's an honorable record."

"It's an honorable record!" He mimicked my voice. "Ask the gentiles."

"Well, it's time they knew it."

"The *Communist Manifesto* was written a hundred years ago, *nicht wahr?* Has anti-Semitism declined at all?"

"Prejudices die slowly."

"Slowly, slowly," he said. "That is what you Social Democrats always preach."

Saul, the butcher, violently disagreed with Aaron (Orthodox Jews were no Zionists). A fine big man with a graying beard, he had become one of my patients. Butchers are good patients.

"Aaron is a nut," he said. "Zionism, Zionism, Zionism—he tried to convert people even in temple. We are told that one day the Messiah will come and lead all the Jews, living and dead, to the Promised Land. Aaron says, 'Now!' I ask you, *Herr Doktor,* if you had the choice of being led to Eretz Yisroel by the Messiah *or Aaron,* which one would you take?" He whacked off a chunk of meat.

"But also something is wrong with him up here." And with his wounded right forefinger Saul pointed to his forehead. "Do you know that he will not walk one step beyond the bridge over the Wulka? When we were kids we often tried to pull him beyond it. He would yell and scream in a fit, until his mother came rushing to rescue him. You take an occasional walk with him, yes? All right, here is some advice: if he's bothering you too much with all his yap-yap-yapping, walk toward the bridge, fast. Suddenly you will find yourself alone."

I seemed to remember that when Aaron and I walked along the *Judengasse,* which ran to the Wulka, he always stopped before we came to the bridge.

I can see the age-old houses lining the street, each with its little store; Jew Street was the business street of the town. I remember the street in the dawn, as I came from a call, and a line of figures in black on their way toward the synagogue for early-morning services. I see the *bocherim,* the Talmud students, with their wide hats and long sidewhiskers, sedately walking from their dormitory to the school, a yellow baroque building with a beautiful arch. I feel and hear the hustle and bustle on weekdays, peasant carts by the dozen, filled with produce, groaning and rumbling down the street. And now all that is history; before long the new barbarians would come and raze those museum pieces of architecture, the synagogue and the school, and plunder the shops. And where is Aaron, who told me about the barbarians of old?

Perhaps most vividly I remember Purim, the highlight of the year, the anniversary of the great event when Esther, the Persian king's wife, persuaded him to spare her people's lives. Instead of killing the Jews he ordered the execution of the evil Haman, his prime minister. On the eve of Purim the story was read in synagogue, and every time the worshipers heard the name Haman, they stamped on the old wooden floor.

The next day was *the* day. A small stage was built in the middle of Jew Street. It was my first *Purimspiel,* and I asked what the stage was for. "For the *bocherim,*" I was told. "They are the actors in the play." Those pale youngsters who walked with heads bowed were going to act? Then the play would be a very solemn one indeed. Little did I know! On Purim everything is permitted; the holy grayness of synagogue and school changes to uninhibited joy, and one can poke fun at everybody, not excluding the Chief Rabbi himself.

I stood with Aaron at his window, looking down on the stage. A boy wearing the cap and bells of a jester came bouncing onto the stage and chanted the prologue. Then someone in a great fur coat appeared, the image of Herr Weiner, the wealthiest man in town. With him came a pretty young girl (a *bocher,* of course, dressed in girl's clothes)—quite as it should be, because Herr Weiner was known as an admirer of the opposite sex. He stroked the girl's face and pinched her bottom. A gale of laughter swept through Jew Street. Herr Weiner and the damsel disappeared. There was a pause.

And *I* walked on stage.

No question about it. I walked just as I walked, and I carried my doctor's bag. All eyes turned up to the window where I stood with Aaron. The other Dr. Berczeller placed my bag on a table. He took out a stethoscope and a tongue depressor. A trembling patient appeared. "Open your mouth. Say 'Ah.' Wider. Good. I can see. Yes, I see them clearly."

"Glug, glug. Wh-wh-wh-what do you see?"

"Your inflamed tonsils. Gargle with peroxide. Aspirin four times a day. Four times a day. Four times a day. Four times a day."

"Four times a day?"

"Four times a day. I hate to repeat myself! Four times a day."

"But *Herr Doktor*—"

"Well? What? Speak up!"

"Do you have a longer stick than the one you put in my mouth?"

"A longer stick! Why?"

"Because I want you to look up the other end. I have a bad case of piles."

Again there was laughter in Jew Street. The doctor and his patient trotted away.

A tall, dignified man in caftan came next—the rabbi, of course, followed by a *bocher* (an Orthodox rabbi never walks without escort).

"Worthy Rabbi, I have a problem. Why is it cold in winter and hot in summer?"

The imitation rabbi slowly stroked his imitation beard. "Very simple. In winter we heat the stoves, the warm air goes up and stays up until summer, when it comes down. Understand?"

"Yes, worthy Rabbi. But then why is it cold in winter?"

"Even more simple. Do you notice anybody lighting stoves *in the summer?*"

Great laughter.

And now a small elderly man wearing a helmet climbed the steps to the stage. I glanced at the small elderly man in his helmet next to me. His face was tense. "It's all in fun," I whispered. The Aaron on the stage took a little blue and white flag, the Zionist flag, from his pocket and waved it and spoke in the very voice of Aaron. "Fellow Jews! What are we doing in this unfriendly land? Follow me to the land of our ancestors!" And he marched down off the stage and up the street through the crowd until he came to the bridge over the Wulka. There he stopped. He trembled, he shook, he wept. He turned and ran as fast as his feet would carry him.

A shout from the crowd: "Aaron, how are you going to take us to Eretz Yisroel if you can't get across that damned bridge?"

Huge laughter.

Aaron was no longer at my side. I went downstairs. There he was, bent over the ancient press. "Don't take it to heart," I said. He shrugged.

Beyond all doubt he was a case of agoraphobia. In that mo-

ment it seemed to me that the Wulka creek was also the historic
dividing line between the ghetto and the gentile world. Wasn't
Aaron's agoraphobia his fear of passing into that hostile world?
I didn't watch the rest of the spectacle.

To translate the word *Fasching* as "carnival" is a purely liter-
ary exercise, having little if any connection with reality. Worries,
disputes, even political antagonism, especially violent in the Austria of the 1930s, were put off, or anyway held down somewhat,
until February, when the *Fasching* season ended. It was celebrated by the thousands of groups and societies in which Austria
was so abundant. Shoemakers, carpenters, plumbers, postal clerks,
mechanics, chimney sweeps, stonemasons, peasants, all celebrated
with music and dancing and drinking in countless inns all over
the country, night after night.

And so, naturally, for a country doctor *Fasching* was an extremely busy time, as he treated the wounds caused by beer mugs
flying through the air.

Late one February night my bell rang. I looked out the window. A peasant cart stood below. The driver spoke. *"Kummans,
Herr Dokta.* It is a matter of life and death."

I dressed and hurried down. He was an innkeeper from Rohr-
bach, a village ten kilometers away, and I was the nearest doctor.
"Don't take your car," he advised. "The roads are frozen fast."

I got into the cart. Herr Kutrowatz clucked at the horse. I had
never been to his inn, the Black Bull. "A fight over a girl," he
said. "Her sweetheart got angry when another boy asked her for a
dance. *Si wissens ja eh.* Who is sober at two in the morning? A
wine bottle broke. The boy is bleeding."

The trip took us more than an hour. Inside the Black Bull a
boy of about twenty lay in a puddle of blood. He was dead; the
broken glass had severed a tributary of the carotid artery. The
kerosene lamp dangling from the ceiling made the silent, watching
faces seem as pale as the dead boy's. A girl had the corner of her

dirndl apron over her face. Next to her stood a boy with large
frightened red-rimmed eyes.

Two police officers arrived and questioned Herr Kutrowatz.
"Who threw the bottle?"

"*Ich weiss nicht,*" he said with a shrug.

"Then who was it?"

Silence.

"Do you have any idea, *Herr Doktor?*"

"No," I said.

The officer snapped his notebook shut. "Hopeless," he said.
"I've been in this section for twenty years, and I can't remember a
single time when I was successful in investigating a *Wirtshaus-
rauferei.*"

The cart hobbled and groaned along the awful road. The
night, or very early morning, the hour just before dawn, seemed
more bitterly cold than any I could remember, and I made up my
mind to buy a fur-lined coat.

"Young people, hot blood," Herr Kutrowatz said. "Jealous
boys, pretty girls. The main thing is, the *Obrigkeit* must be kept
out."

He looked at me sideways. "When he asked you that question,
I held my breath."

"What question?"

" 'Do you have any idea, *Herr Doktor?*' Of course you knew,
didn't you?"

"Yes."

"You're a regular guy, *Herr Doktor,* as we plain people say."

Mattersburg was the county seat. The administrative officials
and judges and lawyers, along with some retired military officers
and their wives, made up the local elite. Their club was the Deut-
scher Gesangverein. We were not invited to any of their affairs,
in which I was profoundly uninterested—and where would I
have found the time to go? But Maria resented not being asked.

"Where are we going to find friends? The Orthodox Jews? The peasants?"

"I hope you don't give a damn for any of the Gesangverein nincompoops."

"I don't. But is it right for us to spend our young lives here?"

"Vienna's only an hour and a half away."

I knew her answer to that: half a year had passed since my last visit to Vienna. We had season's tickets for the opera and concerts, but just as we were about to get into the Opel, something would come up. During the last visit we went to a performance of *Lohengrin,* and in the middle of the crescendo from the orchestra that would have stirred the dead, I uttered a snore. And—Maria would continue—I even neglected my postgraduate courses. We would stay in Mattersburg to the ends of our lives, as Dr. Klinger had. And one day Peter would go to the three-hundred-year-old Jewish public school, with classes into which three grades were squeezed.

The last, of course, was the most powerful part of her argument. I was growing to know it very well.

⊰ *xiv* ⊱

"WHY IS YOUR SONG SO SAD?"

Peter was fed according to the latest principles, which in those days were still the ancient ones: breast-feeding. I can hear his loud gulps; I can see Maria's solemn face, and their eyes looking earnestly at each other. She seemed more his older sister than his mother. He was weighed before and after each feeding; if he weighed a little less than expected, she behaved as though doom were just around the corner.

Little by little, breast-feeding changed to mixed-feeding; grated carrot and minced spinach and other valuable substances went into his mouth, and how he grew! How his teeth developed! And how he spoke! How he stood upright, on his very own feet! That was what Maria pointed out to me. "Look! He stands on his very own, his *very own* feet!"

"Whose else would they be?" I asked.

One day when I came in he staggered toward me like an affectionate drunk. His first real suit was a Tyrolean *Janker* and shorts, which he wore with a Tyrolean hat with feather. (We later lost most of our possessions as we fled across Europe, but we still have a little picture of Peter in his Tyrolean hat.) The front seat of the car was *his* seat. He knew all the bumps in the country roads and would warn me in advance. *"Jessas, der Peter!"* the women in the villages exclaimed as we drove past and Peter waved—a strong, healthy little boy with a tanned face. The Viennese children all seemed pale.

Another winter came, bringing with it the usual respiratory illnesses. In Mattersburg things went relatively well, but in Forchtenau, only a few kilometers away, fifteen people died of pneumonia. In the foothills of the Rosalia Mountains, Forchtenau enjoyed an excellent climate and was famous for its sturdy citizens. Why was there such a disproportionate mortality? The Forchtenau doctor had been well trained at a Viennese hospital and had done everything to find the reason; he had sent the patients' sputa and blood to a Vienna laboratory. As was only to be expected, not one of them would agree to be transferred to a hospital: people were cut up in hospitals and died.

One day I was called to Forchtenau for consultation. The wealthiest fruit-grower, Herr Halder, was desperately ill. He had begun to sneeze and cough two weeks ago, but of course had gone on with his work as usual. Then his temperature rose and rose, and for the first time in his life he couldn't work.

Do young doctors today see those classical four stages of the disease, once so dreaded; the numerous post mortems, the red or gray "hepatization"? How helpless we were! I see myself standing at the sickbed; I hear myself prescribing cough medicines and recommending a good hot bowl of chicken soup and cold compresses for the fever, digitalis when the heart failed, a camphor injection. . . .

Herr Halder was indeed ill, breathing laboriously. He had lobar pneumonia. I retired with my colleague, Dr. Löffler, to discuss the case. Basically there was nothing to discuss.

Eight or nine days later old Halder's son turned up in my waiting-room, looking cheerful. I couldn't believe my eyes. Surely his father was dead.

He shook my hand warmly. "Heartfelt thanks, *Herr Doktor!*"

"How is your father?" I asked.

"*Pumperlgesund!*"

I must have gaped at him.

"*Ja!*" he said. "Let me tell you! We didn't have much hope, God knows, but then you came with that machine. First you placed a kind of cuff around his arm and pumped air into it. The cuff got swollen and then slowly went down again, while you watched a kind of little clock. From that moment my father felt better. Better isn't the word!" Young Halder laughed, and I ventured to join him. "The next morning he ate Paprika Speck and drank a *Stamperl,* the very same breakfast he's eaten for as long as I can remember. He feeds the pigs as usual, *Herr Doktor,* and prunes the fruit trees, and to you he sends his very best regards."

The young man took out his wallet and put a hundred-schilling bill in my hand. I could not refrain at that moment from glancing at my blood-pressure apparatus.

Work in minor surgery was abundant. I remember the case of a farmer who stumbled over his scythe, cutting his right arm from the shoulder blade to the hand, a gaping wound that exposed the muscles and nerves; some of the muscles were partially severed. During my Krankenhaus der Stadt Wien days such a case was treated by either the professor or one of his assistants.

The patient, Herr Lehner, looked at me with astonishment when I suggested that he might prefer to go to the hospital. "But *Herr Doktor, der Herr Doktor* Klinger would have done it himself!"—at least that was what his eyes seemed to say. I warned him that some of the nerves might have been severed and if he was not treated properly his hand might be partially or even totally paralyzed. "*Machen Sie es!*" he said and waved agreeably with his other hand.

He had arrived around noon; until the late afternoon I worked on him, putting in stitch after stitch. I had a little peasant-girl nurse by then, but she was still liable to fainting spells at the sight of nasty wounds, so I had called Maria to assist me. Her face became paler and paler as she watched, and dainty pearls appeared on her forehead. I sent her away to join my nurse.

As for Herr Lehner, he did not faint! "You need help, *Herr Doktor?*" he asked.

"Well—" I said.

"Good," he said. "My left hand is still working."

I scrubbed his left hand. Sitting on the operating-room chair he handed me needles and pincers and so on, meanwhile watching curiously. There was no pain because of the local anesthetic. *"Sehr gut, Herr Doktor,"* he said in commendation after I had applied the final dressing. Maria still mentions this case once in a while: the patient who helped.

Things did not always work out so smoothly. One of Ferdl's neighbors came to the office with his wife. He had fallen from a tall tree and probably would have been killed if a strong lower branch hadn't caught him. His abdomen hurt. Examining him, I felt a mass behind the umbilicus that grew in size by the second. The diagnosis was not difficult: a hematoma caused by internal hemorrhage. I advised immediate hospitalization.

"Nein, nein," he said. "People die in hospitals."

"That isn't true. You must go at once."

"For such a trifle? No."

"You will die if you don't."

"If I must die, I prefer to die at home." He smiled at his wife, who nodded.

A few hours later he was dead. Two days after that I watched the funeral procession, led by the veterans' band.

I drove up to Burg Forchtenstein to talk to Ferdl. "It was not my fault," I said. "I couldn't force him to go to the hospital. All the same, I can't help thinking about it—the young wife, now a widow, and the children."

"Forget it," Ferdl said. "He would have died even if he'd gone to the hospital, and his wife would have blamed it on you and the hospital for the rest of her life. They just won't go to hospitals."

They just won't go to hospitals. I often wondered how Dr. Klinger had acted in cases of abdominal emergency. I could not ask him, and the tombstones in the cemetery were mute.

Peter spent every second or third weekend with his grandparents. Father's offices were now in Eisenstadt, seventeen kilometers away. I would walk hand-in-hand with Peter through the narrow crooked streets of the old town and show him the little house with geranium pots on the window sills where Franz Josef Haydn had lived, then up to the magnificent baroque castle of the Dukes of Esterházy and the *Musiksaal* with frescoes on the walls. On that same platform, I explained, Haydn himself had sat at the piano. We strolled through the gardens, which reminded me of Versailles and the Trianon, and at last came to the baroque church, the so-called Haydn-church, with the tomb of the maestro. Who could add anything to the five letters?

H A Y D N

In Father's office Peter sat in his chair and played with colored crayons, just as my grandchildren now sit in my office chair and play with colored crayons. A few years ago Peter visited Eisenstadt. When he returned to New York he said he had looked at the same chair and, as though in a haze, that long-ago time came back to him—even the crayons. But someone else was sitting there.

People were kind to *Frau Doktor* Berczeller. As always happens, I suppose—at least with country doctors—the patients feel that the doctor's wife must also know a good deal of what the doctor knows, and if they felt dissatisfied with me, they would leave my office and repair to the living room or the kitchen and tell Maria their problems. Frau Handler took a special liking to her. *"Sie ist eine fesche Frau, und gescheit,"* the old lady said to me when we met professionally. (She had become reconciled with Ferdl, now her grandson-in-law; once when I passed his house I saw her blacking his boots.) She was an almost daily visitor to the doctor's apartment in a nonprofessional capacity. A midwife knows all the town's secrets, and she passed them on to Maria, who, it must be remembered, although the mother of a fine son, was still not much more than a girl. Occasionally I would reap the benefit of this behind-the-scenes knowledge, as when Maria solemnly informed me about the progress of Frau Pinter's love affair with August, the handsome carpenter. "It will come to no good end," she predicted.

One night at dinner she gave me a stern look. "You don't seem to know what's going on around you," she observed.

"I don't?"

"No. Frau Handler was here today—"

"Is that so!" I said jokingly. "What a surprise!"

"She told me that Paula is pregnant. *Pregnant!"*

"Who is Paula?"

"You don't know who Paula is? She is Ferdl's new housemaid. *Now* do you understand?"

"No," I said.

"As always, you have a one-track mind. Look at the evidence. One and one make two, don't they? Yes, of course. Well, there are three women in Ferdl's house—Frau Handler, Resl, and Paula, who is young, plump, and, I suppose some people would say, pretty. And," Maria continued with heavy meaning, "only one man: *Ferdl.*"

I thought I was listening to Frau Handler. "He may be the only man in the house," I said, "but is he the only man in the world?" (Now I thought I was listening to Ferdl.)

"He has a nice home and a beautiful little boy. Ah, that *böser Mensch!* With a pretty housemaid around, one can't be sure of one's own husband."

I got a little angry. "Don't be ridiculous. And don't mix in other people's business. Let them handle their own affairs."

"Ha!" she exclaimed. "Let them handle their own affairs, you say? Now, if old Dr. Klinger were still here—"

"That is quite enough! I work like a horse all day, and when I come home at night I'm supposed to worry about Paula? And Frau Handler? And Resl? Leave me alone!"

She retired, and I heard a sob from the kitchen. In consequence I didn't sleep well. The next morning I drove up the winding road. Ferdl was cleaning his rifle at the door. "Hey, *Herr Doktor!*" he shouted. "Come in and have a glass or two!"

A new terrace had been added to the house, and we sat down there. "Paula," Ferdl called, "get us a bottle from the cellar, vintage '12."

In a few minutes Paula appeared, middle-sized, with blue eyes and pigtails, a pretty village lass. *"Guten Morgen, Herr Doktor,"* she greeted me with a smile, putting down the bottle. The lower part of her abdomen was distinctly swollen under the dirndl. I looked at it and looked at Ferdl.

He laughed. "Not this time, *Herr Doktor!* You can draw all the blood you want, but you can't make me the father! *Prosit!*"

It was the time of the chestnut harvest, and the air was filled with their fragrance. The giant chestnuts of Forchtenau are famous all over Austria. My colleague in the village was off on vacation, and I filled in for him, usually taking Peter with me. After my calls we wandered around among the peasant houses— nothing very special. Then my eyes caught sight of a house unlike any other, a tiny baroque building with flowers all around the entrance and in pots on the window sills. The house was called the *Fürstenhof,* I learned, because the administrator of the Duke of Esterházy's estates had lived in it with his family. We heard the sound of a piano—a Schubert *Lied,* I thought. The music drew me closer. I stopped. Presently the front door opened, and a young woman looked at us and smiled.

"Ah, you must be the *Herr Doktor* Berczeller," she said. "And this must be Peter. Won't you come in for a visit?"

She wasn't a young woman; her hair was white. The clear, unlined face and youthful eyes had deceived me.

"Thank you," I said. "And you are—"

"Mida Huber, music teacher."

We entered a small, typical baroque room, with a piano near the window. Many sketches and drawings, of houses, people, gardens, decorated the walls. "Drawing is my hobby," she explained.

I told her I wished she would continue with the Schubert. "It is far from Schubert!" she said with a laugh. "My own work, such as it is." She sat down at the piano. If the piece was not Schubert, it was very close.

Occasionally she came to my office for minor troubles, and sometimes I saw her in the ghetto, sketching. "Just look at that building," she would say, "crumbling to pieces, yet still so much grandeur."

The years passed, and the decades. The other day a small package came to me from the Burgenland. In it there was a photograph of a very old lady with large youthful eyes; there were also a few drawings of the long-vanished ghetto and a page of music and words, and a letter. The letter read:

> *Hochgeehrter Herr Doktor!*
> Through diligent inquiries I found your address in New York, as you see! Forgive my almost unreadable handwriting —in April I will be ninety. Please regard my letter as an expression of my prayer still to live a bit [*Ausdruck von ein bisschen Lebenswillen*]. Here is my "Schubert" song. The words—well, poetry was also one of my wrongdoings. How is little Peter? What a big man he must be by now.

The words:

ARMER SPIELMAN

Spielmann, sag warum dein Lied so traurig klingt
Und kein lustig Stücklein dir, aus den Saiten springt?
Komm, spiel uns zum Tanze auf, trink ein Krügel Wein!
Jag hinweg die Traurigkeit, wird dir wohler sein!
Möcht schon gerne trinken, doch vom Born, der im Walde
*   quillt,*
Der vergessen bringen soll und das Herzweh stillt.
Wo mag nur der Brunnen sein klar wie grünes Licht?
Irre schon so lang umher, doch ich fand ihn nicht.
Ich fand ihn nicht.

Freely translated,

Minstrel man, why is your song so sad?
From your strings please pluck a cheerful note!
A song to dance to! Come, drink a glass of wine!
Banish your sorrow! Drink, minstrel man!

I wish I could drink, from a spring deep in the woods,
Which would let me forget, and soothe my heartache.
Where is that spring, clear as green light?
I wander and wander, but I cannot find it.
I cannot find it.

THE VANISHING TRIMMEL

Often during the dark winter months of 1930 and 1931, I thought of Professor Grassberger and his lectures on hygiene. "Cleanliness, *meine Herren!* That is the only secret, the only way to avoid epidemics! Cleanliness, cleanliness, cleanliness! Remember!"

In the intervals between his quotations from Cicero, Sophocles, and others, and his references to the Crusades and the French Revolution ("As for me, I would have been a Girondist; Charlotte Corday was right!"), he spoke about typhoid fever and how to avoid it. His *Hochquellenwasserleitung* was part of the answer, along with cleanliness, but sporadic cases still turned up. Peasant women carried milk diluted with water in open containers from the country to Vienna, and occasionally the water came from wells into which excrement had seeped from outdoor toilets, carrying the typhoid bacillus. Some people who had recovered from the illness remained, unwittingly, typhoid carriers: their stools contained the bacilli, harmless to the host but very much alive and all too often deadly for others.

Typhoid was endemic in Mattersburg and the surrounding villages. I do not recall a single month during my years of country practice when I did not see a typhoid case. Once in a while it flared up into epidemic proportions. That was what happened in the winter of 1930 and 1931.

Early in November I was called by a farmer to examine his son, a young man of twenty. Cough, fever, abdominal distress were the symptoms; temperature, 43 Celsius, *râles* over the lungs. My first impression was of pneumonia; but then, examining the abdomen, I discovered the well-known pink spots around the umbilicus, and a slightly elevated spleen; he also had a "dicrotic" pulse (slow, compared with the high temperature): typhoid fever.

A second, a third, a fourth case developed . . . and a thirtieth. There seemed to be no end; call after call after call I saw the same symptoms, by now so familiar. The shutters of the sickrooms were always meticulously closed, as though to keep out further harm. I can see those dark, low-ceilinged rooms; I can smell the damp, unclean air. Worst of all was the tension of waiting: three, four, five, sometimes six weeks would pass before one knew—life or death. The days shadowed into nights, the nights into days. My dreams were filled with horror. Once, I remember, I was fighting bubonic plague and writing my epitaph, and standing with Liesl, embracing her near a tomb on which, lo and behold, the name was my own.

Why had I left Vienna and come to this cursed place?

Maria's Mohnstrudels, expertly prepared by now, lost their taste. I had no appetite at all. My only desire was to sleep. Then I reached the stage where sleep was impossible. One night I turned over and back and over again in bed until two in the morning. Maria slept like a baby—like Peter, blissfully slumbering! I got up, walked quietly from the room, went to my office: scores of medical magazines and unopened envelopes—I had no time to read. I thought I would catch up a little, but before I could settle down with a new medical journal I saw a very old one, a very old book, the book with the flowers on the cover, Dr. Ziffer's contribution to medical knowledge. What did *he* have to say about typhoid fever? I looked in the index under the letter T.

> *Tetük* [lice]
> *Tojás* [eggs]
> *Tornázás* [gymnastics]
> *Tyúkszem* [corn]

Under the letter T there was no mention whatever of typhoid fever.

I looked under the letter F: fevers, but no typhoid.

But this was impossible. Western medicine's knowledge of typhoid went back to the 1820s. Perhaps Dr. Ziffer had forgotten to list it in the index? Perhaps the editors or the typesetters were at fault? I leafed through the pages devoted to the letter T. I read about the anatomy, the physiology, the pathology of lice. I read Dr. Ziffer's learned remarks about the form, content, and the recommended ways of cooking eggs (you can boil them, you can fry them, you can poach them, you can bake them; they are *extremely nutritious*). No typhoid fever. Writing in the 1860s, with typhoid all around him, perhaps Dr. Ziffer thought—as others have thought about other grave matters—that if he ignored typhoid fever, it would go away.

The epidemic slowly petered out, after taking its toll: dozens of new graves of the old, the middle-aged, the young, the very young.

Fortunately there was a change from the winter's grim routine. Something happened to me which sounds like grist for a wildly farcical movie, but I swear by Hippocrates it was true.

The colonel stood out among the patients in my waiting-room, a distinguished figure in breeches and high boots, his snow-white hair stiffly brushed back, a riding-crop in one hand. When I entered the room, he jumped to his feet and clicked his heels.

"Oberst im Ruhestand [retired colonel] von Weidinger!" he said crisply. We shook hands.

While walking in his yard he had fallen and hurt his left arm and wrist. Someone told him that I had an X-ray machine, and he had come to learn if there was a fracture. The film showed none; it was only a sprain. I gave him the indicated advice; he thanked me and asked for the bill. "Thirty schillings," I said.

"Thirty schillings, *Herr Doktor?* Not enough! Fifty!"

"Thirty is quite enough, *Herr Oberst.*"

Without another word he took out three ten-shilling notes. In his gray eyes I thought I could read: Here is a decent chap.

A few days later, driving up a mountain road, I heard someone call, *"Herr Doktor, Herr Doktor."* It was the *Herr Oberst,* in khaki shirt and wide peasant hat but still in gleaming boots and with riding-crop in hand. "Can you stop for a few minutes?" he asked. I discovered that this visit was not so much to see how his arm and wrist were progressing as for a chat.

We crossed a wide yard surrounded by a chicken-wire fence. Hundreds, or perhaps thousands, of chickens occupied this compound. A majestic rooster, lord of the realm, marched around with short firm steps, and I thought of a lancer on sentry-go. There were henhouses in the background.

"My chicken farm," the *Herr Oberst* said. He might as well have said, "The parade ground."

He lived in a hut. Inside, I saw a cot, an unpolished table, two chairs, a bookcase containing four or five books (I could imagine their contents), and pictures of various generals. The largest picture was of Emperor Franz Josef; another, not quite so large, of Conrad von Hötzendorf, chief of staff of the Austro-Hungarian Army in the late war.

The air smelled of boot polish and pipe tobacco. "Please sit down, *Herr Doktor,"* my host said. He stepped to a chest in one corner and came back with a bottle of champagne. He poured two glasses. *"Prosit!* And, as a toast, something my mother always said in times of disaster: *'In allem schlechten ist etwas gut!'* How right she was! In anything bad, something good is hidden. That tumble of mine brought me to you, *Herr Doktor."*

We took our glasses outside and sat on a bench. It was one of those March days when the sun is warm but the mountain wind freezing. The colonel puffed on an English pipe and asked if I had time for another glass of champagne. I couldn't refuse; eventually we emptied the bottle.

I had a long list of patients to visit, and when I finally got to them they must have thought the doctor was in quite a jolly mood.

After that, I stopped quite often at the chicken farm. "What gave you the idea of starting it, *Herr Oberst?"* I asked one day.

"Quite simple, really. My wife died of the Spanish flu during the war. She had always bought our eggs from a chicken farm in the district because, she said, the chickens were expertly fed and looked after, and in consequence the eggs were delicious. After the war I was placed on the retired list—how many colonels were needed in the new dwarf-sized Austrian Army? And in any event I would never have served in the Army of the Republic. My pension was small; I had to supplement it. How? At sixty what could I do? A bookkeeper? Anything involving mathematics is anathema to me. I remembered my wife's remarks about the eggs. Ha! An acre of ground in the country, a few henhouses, a few hens, a good rooster, and let nature take its course. You see the result, *Herr Doktor."*

"They multiply easily."

"Indeed they do. And something else; have you ever seen chickens coming out of their little houses when the doors are opened? No? Like young recruits rushing from the barracks for their breakfast! Swift, lively, full of strength and movement!

Good soldiers-to-be!" The colonel puffed on his pipe. One corner of his mouth was slightly elevated. It could have been the barest token of a smile.

"So I searched for the right location. The closer you are to Vienna, the more expensive it is. I came here. Fresh mountain air—good for me, good for my recruits!" And now there was really a smile under the short white mustache.

"Then you are happy, *Herr Oberst.*"

"Happy? Well, as close as I could come to it in times like these. One lives in the past. Good God, how people have changed! There is no discipline, there is no respect for one's neighbor. In a word, *Herr Doktor,* we live in a world of common people."

I ventured to disagree.

"Common people, *Herr Doktor!* You know it as well as I, but your nature forbids you to say so. Never mix with them if you can help it. Mother used to say, 'If you fall into the swill, the pigs will eat you.' Again, how right she was! It is especially true of these Burgenland people. Even if you're from a neighboring town, they regard you as a suspicious foreigner. If you come from Vienna, beware! Oh, yes, to your face they are kind, even submissive, but behind your back—my God, what won't they say, the damnedest lies and nonsense!"

"They've been very kind to me, *Herr Oberst.*"

"Purely selfishness; they need your services. But a chicken-farmer, he is a competitor."

Of course I didn't agree with these sentiments, but after all, what else could one expect from a former *Kaiserlich und Königlicher* officer, an aristocrat? I thought of ash-blond Liesl and her father; it seemed to me it would be pleasant to see General Rüdiger Count von Hohengraben as a chicken farmer.

April arrived with soft, warm winds. On my visits the *Herr Oberst* would bring out a bottle of *Gumpoldskirchner,* a dry white wine from the Vienna hills, and tell stories about the war. He had been on the Russian front in the bleak winter of 1914 and 1915, a time he would never forget, with the catastrophic retreat of our army over the Carpathian Mountains and down into the Fatherland itself. With the handle of his riding-crop he drew diagrams—arrows pointing this way and that, with holes scooped in the earth to illustrate various hazards. Occasionally a stray chicken wandered across the field of battle.

"Now, here is the army column of General Auffenberg," the *Herr Oberst* said, "and here is a second column commanded by General Dankl. On the offensive, they marched straight toward the plains of Polish Russia and even occupied Lublin. What they forgot was that the Russians were not *aufs Hirn gefallen* either." He tapped his forehead. "The Grand Duke Nicholas, the Czar's uncle, was their commander, and, I must admit, a crafty one. He permitted us to march into a trap. Hundreds of thousands of our men died in that wasteland of snow, and, later, in the Carpathians. Other hundreds of thousands were taken prisoner. In my opinion, that disaster decided the whole war. That it was, incidentally, the beginning of the end for the Romanovs was a poor consolation for us Austrians. I do not indulge in self-pity, *Herr Doktor*, but once in a while I am bound to admit that I feel— Well, consider. When the war began I was a captain; three years later, a colonel. Just a little longer, and I would have been promoted to brigadier general. Still, why should I complain?" And his face brightened as he pointed at the army of chickens.

Other famous battles and campaigns were sketched out for me in the dirt by the colonel's riding-crop. "We and the Germans would have beaten the whole lot of them if the United States hadn't intervened at the very end. President Wilson and his infamous fourteen points!" he said. *"Betrug!"*

My telephone rang. The commander of the local police was on the wire. I hardly recognized his voice, he was so excited. "Please, *Herr Doktor*, come as soon as you can! Come at once!" Bang went the receiver, before I could ask what was wrong.

The police station was at the other end of town. There was a crowd at the entrance. It greeted me respectfully and cleared a path. Inside, the commander's stocky, plump figure, with ruddy face, typical of an officer who has come up through the ranks, positively jumped out of his chair. "As long as I've been here, almost twenty-five years, never anything like this—never!" he shouted.

"What is it?" I asked.

"You'll see!"

In the small room behind his office I saw something completely unexpected—the colonel. He sat quite at ease, smoking his English pipe. The gleaming boots were on his feet, the riding-crop was in his hand; all was as usual, but he was wrapped in a coarse blanket. He clutched it to him as he sprang up. *"Guten Morgen, Herr Doktor!"* he said cheerfully.

I turned to the police commander. "Please tell me what this is all about."

"Herr Doktor, I heard women screaming, men's shouts, an uproar! In came one of my men, holding the *Herr Oberst's* arm. *Herr Doktor,* I say it to my regret, it deeply distresses me to say it, but it must be said. The *Herr Oberst, Herr Doktor,* was naked. He was stark naked, *Herr Doktor,* except for his boots."

"Quite so," the colonel said in an unconcerned voice. "Boots, certainly."

I looked at him; he smiled. "But why, *Herr Oberst?"* I asked.

"Quite simple," he replied. "Let me tell you the course of events—that is, if you can spare a few minutes?" He looked at me inquiringly, I nodded, and he sat down. "I have mentioned the disrespectful, not to say prying and sneaking, behavior of the local people—no regard whatsoever for a former imperial officer, even among veterans of the war. Lately it has grown worse. I heard them whispering behind me when I came to town to buy supplies for the farm. 'He does not feed his chickens,' they whispered. 'Even though they are only birds, one must pity the poor little souls. The *Herr Oberst* is stingy. What a shame.' I felt like giving them a good thrashing with my riding-crop but held myself back; after all, it would have been beneath my dignity. But this morning something happened which I absolutely could not ignore. I was bound to respond, *Herr Doktor*."

"What happened?"

"I heard two men behind me. 'Look at him,' said one, 'thin as a shadow. He starves his chickens, he starves himself.' The other chipped in. 'I'll bet even his'—a certain private part—'is thin as a needle.' That was enough. I slowly undressed and let them see for themselves. Of course I kept my boots on. I have worn them since I was a cadet."

There was a short silence.

"Today—today," the police commander stammered, "weekly market day! Hundreds of women in the street, *Herr Doktor!* Perhaps you can visualize the stir among them?"

By now I had regained my presence of my mind. I remembered my first psychiatric patient. *"Herr Oberst,"* I said, "I understand your indignation; the behavior of some of these country people is intolerable. Let me see if something can't be done about it. Excuse me for a few minutes." I made a sign to the commander, who followed me out of the room. "Is there a phone I can use?"

"There, *Herr Doktor*. What do you intend to do?"

"I am going to call a friend of mine at the psychiatric hospital in Vienna."

Before long I had him on the phone—Dr. Hammer, a classmate and good friend. I told him the colonel's story. "Clear as sunshine," he said. "Paranoid schizophrenic, as of course you must have realized. For a while he dissimulated, as they all do, then finally broke out, *nicht wahr?*"

"Well?" I said. "We can't keep him here."

"Send him to us. We'll admit him."

"Then you send an ambulance here."

"An ambulance?" Hammer said. "Are you crazy? Do you mean

to say you've forgotten how hard it is to send an ambulance beyond the city limits? We'd get so tangled up in red tape it wouldn't be there for a week. Tell me, is your *Herr Oberst* violent?"

"Not in the least; he is a perfectly well-controlled man."

"Well, then, send him to us by train, accompanied by some reliable person. Why not come yourself, *alter Tepp,* and we'll have a night out, eh?"

"You don't know how how busy I am."

I relayed Hammer's suggestion to the police commander. Frowning, he scratched his head and then nodded. "Trimmel is the man, absolutely reliable. You remember him, *Herr Doktor,* he came to you with a sore finger."

I remembered Trimmel—thirty-five or so, about the colonel's height, six feet, well built, a police sergeant and a veteran of the Imperial Army. The colonel would have plenty of material to discuss with him.

Trimmel came to the office, and I explained the case, warning him that there was, as in all psychiatric cases, a possibility of non-cooperation, but, I thought, a very remote one. Everything should go smoothly.

"Whatever happens, *Herr Doktor,* I'll be able to handle it, don't worry," Trimmel said. He was very cheerful, and I was sure I understood why. A free ride to Vienna, a day off? I was the one who had the unpleasant job: explaining things to the colonel.

I returned to the little room. "We are going to find those two *Tunichguts* who insulted you, *Herr Oberst,* and teach them a lesson. But it has been a trying experience for you, also these stupid country people are still babbling their heads off, and in my opinion you should have a rest until things calm down. I've just spoken with two friends of mine in Vienna, a retired major and his wife. They have asked you to spend a few days with them."

"Very kind," the colonel said, "and I would like to. But who will take care of the farm?"

"That was the first thing I thought of. I phoned the mayor of Forchtenau, a patient of mine, and he says he knows another chicken-farmer, with an excellent reputation, who will look after things. Nothing to worry about."

"Good!" The colonel took off the blanket and began to dress. He and Trimmel left on the late morning train.

The following morning I had a call from the police commander. "Have you heard from Trimmel?"

"No," I said.

"He hasn't reported back. No reason for alarm; he is absolutely reliable. Perhaps he had a couple of glasses of wine and decided to spend the night away from wife and children." He laughed. "Well, I was young once myself. He'll be here on the afternoon train."

At ten that night the commander did not sound so cheerful when he called. "Trimmel is still not here. *Herr Doktor,* will you call your friend at the psychiatric hospital? It is possible that they never even got there."

I called the hospital at once. Fortunately Hammer was on night duty. "Certainly the patient and escort arrived," he said. "I gave the escort a note saying he had safely delivered the patient. By the way, I've a bone to pick with you, *alter Tepp.* You called him perfectly well controlled, didn't you? This teaches me once again never to trust anyone who isn't a psychiatrist. The perfectly well-controlled patient kicked me in the groin."

"He must have grown suspicious," I said. "I gave him a cock-and-bull story about a friendly major and wife with whom he was going to stay. Sorry."

I called the police commander and gave him Hammer's report. "Well, nothing to do but wait for the morning train," he said. "Damn it, I'm disappointed in Trimmel."

The next morning he was back on the phone. *"Herr Doktor,* still no Trimmel. I must confess I am seriously worried. I've told the Vienna police to investigate—discreetly, of course. Honestly, I cannot help feeling the *Herr Oberst* should have been sent to Vienna by ambulance in the first place."

Three days after Trimmel's disappearance his wife came to my office. If she hadn't come, I would have asked her in for a talk, to learn what I could about their life together, Trimmel's habits, and so on. She was a pretty brunette, dressed like a city woman, as her Viennese accent at once proclaimed her to be.

"I'm almost out of my mind, *Herr Doktor!* Oh my God, what has happened to him? Do you have any idea?"

"I have every confidence in your husband," I said. "But I would like to ask one or two questions. Do you mind?"

"Anything to bring Johann back! Our little son is asking, 'where is Papa?' And the baby girl cries."

"Can your marriage be called a good one, Frau Trimmel?"

"Certainly!"

"Never any arguments about—well, about other women?"

"I should say not! Nothing like that, *Herr Doktor,* ever! If he has a fault, it is that occasionally he will go over his normal two glasses of wine and become a little—a little—" She looked for a word. "A little foolish. But what man isn't, once in a while?"

"Never any morbid talk?"

"Morbid talk?"

"Feeling depressed, perhaps, and mentioning suicide?"

"My God, no!" she exclaimed. "With all his love for the children?"

"And he is in good health?"

"You should know, *Herr Doktor.*"

"All I treated was his sore finger."

"That is the only thing that has ever been wrong with him."

At this point she broke down, and I felt increasingly conscience-stricken. I should not have entrusted a psychopath to a lay person. On the other hand, it was Hammer, a psychiatrist, who had suggested it, and he was always dealing with similar problems. No; if anything had happened to Trimmel (and it certainly seemed that something had), it had come later, had nothing to do with psychiatry.

These rationalizations quieted me down for a while; then more questions came to plague my conscience. Trimmel must have had more than his "normal two glasses" of wine. Well, then, where was he? With an overperfumed professional Viennese lady? Quite a change for a country boy—which was all he was, really.

Had he been murdered?

A nationwide alarm was broadcast for missing Police Sergeant Trimmel. Description: "Six feet, one hundred and eighty-five pounds, ruddy face, blue eyes, dark brown, slightly wavy hair. The missing man smokes Sport cigarettes, speaks German with a Burgenland accent."

When I went on my house calls I thought people looked at me with distinctly less friendly eyes, and it was a fact that there were fewer patients in my waiting-room. Still, it was May, and there was not so much illness. But as I walked along the street, didn't a man turn and glance at me with a frown?

Was *I* now becoming paranoid?

More questions: Were there any secrets in Trimmel's life? A woman? I thought I hit on a clue. As a police sergeant, Trimmel had often driven on a motorbike to surrounding villages, inspecting smaller police posts. Somewhere or other I had heard that he would visit a certain inn, the Black Hound, in the Rosalia Mountains, mostly patronized by backwoods types. It was run by Frau Kerlinger, a widow, who had come to my office for a minor complaint. She was around forty, blond and voluptuous.

I thought I should visit Frau Kerlinger and mention Trimmel's name.

At the Black Hound inn, a young waitress told me that Frau Kerlinger had gone to visit her aunt in Vienna. "How long ago?" I asked.

"Oh, almost three days."

I could have shouted in triumph. "May I have her address, please?"

She gave me the address. I drove home in a jubilant frame of mind. "I have solved it," I announced to Maria.

"You have solved what?"

"The riddle of Trimmel's disappearance. I know precisely where he is."

"Where?"

I told her.

Her face was cool. "So now you are an amateur detective. Why don't you stick to what you know something about?" (To this day I have differences with Maria because of her "lack of enthusiasm.")

The next morning I drove to Vienna, not mentioning my discoveries to the police commander, for fear of raising a hue and cry that would cause Trimmel to bolt. Frau Kerlinger's aunt lived in the Pramergasse, a proletarian district of two- and three-story houses. I walked up three flights with palpitations, not because of the climb but because of the approaching scene, a small drama. The name on the door was the aunt's: Josefine Freiberger. I rang the bell. There was a sound of shuffling steps. Slowly the door opened. The tiny, wrinkled face of a thin old lady looked up at me.

" *Was kann ich für Sie tun?*" she inquired.

"I came to see Frau Kerlinger."

"Come in, please." And the old lady turned and shouted, "Kathy, a gentleman is here to see you." She turned back to me. "She will be here soon, maybe. She needs two hours to wake up, paint her face, and get dressed. You would think she was one of the Vienna *Damen* of high society. What does she do all the time in the woods? She must have enough money by now, *glauben's net?*"

I looked around the small overfurnished room as the old lady babbled on. There was no sign of Trimmel's gray overcoat.

"*Jessas, der Herr Doktor* Berczeller!" someone exclaimed. "*Was für eine Ehre. Was macht mir das Vergnügen—?*"

She seemed pleasantly astonished and somewhat honored to see me. I felt embarrassed. I couldn't start the conversation by blurting out, "Where is Trimmel?"

Fortunately—or perhaps, considering my new, budding career, unfortunately—she took care of the whole matter.

"Just my luck, *Herr Doktor,* not to be at home when for the first time in years there's a real sensation at home. My God, how they all must be talking up at the old Black Hound! That poor Trimmel! A nice fellow, you know—strict, as a policeman has to be, but always absolutely fair. He never came sneaking in the back door to make sure I was closing at midnight. And no bribes, not even a glass of beer on the house. And it had to happen to him. I'm sure he's dead."

"What makes you think so, Frau Kerlinger?"

"Just a guess. Why would a nice fellow like that just disappear?"

The old lady nodded. Then she showed me the kitchen, the bedroom, and the *Kabinett,* as a little nook or den is called in Vienna. "Too big for me." She sighed. "Fine, as long as my poor husband lived. But my good niece comes from time to time, *nicht wahr?*"

"Yes, Aunt."

There was no trace of Trimmel. Frau Kerlinger asked me why I had come by. I made up some kind of story. I was in a deflated mood. My career as an amateur detective had fizzled out. I could imagine Maria's face.

With a little time on my hands, I decided to look in on Hammer. He was making rounds, and I waited an hour in the *Dienstzimmer.*

"You're looking down in the dumps, Richard," he said. "What's wrong?"

"What's wrong?" I said. "What do you think? The famous

affair of the police officer, of course. It's making me miserable."

"What's the trouble with the police officer?"

I looked at him as if he had just arrived from the moon. "The police officer I sent with the schizo—the guard."

"What's he done?" Hammer asked.

"For God's sake, don't you read the papers?"

"If I get time to glance at them, I'm lucky. The chief keeps me over my head in work."

"Do you mean to say you don't know the police-officer guard disappeared after delivering the patient to you? Just as if the earth opened and swallowed him?"

I could see that genuinely astonished Hammer. "*He* disappeared?"

"Without trace."

"But why? Such a responsible-looking man!"

"Who knows why?" I retorted. "All I know is I'm blamed—openly or by implication. The whole town looks at me."

"That's absurd," Hammer said. "You only did what had to be done. Although quite between us, old fellow, you did somewhat misjudge the schizo. Well controlled, you said. You should see him! Like a tiger! His food has to be pushed in through the bars. The toughest wardens won't go near to him when he's having one of his fits."

"Let me have a look at him," I said. "Perhaps if I say 'How are you, *Herr Oberst?*' he'll calm down."

"A colonel already?" Hammer said. "That fellow?"

I was beginning to feel that something was wrong. "Let me see him."

Hammer led me through many doors, then down a corridor. "There he is. Stand well back. I can still feel the kick he gave me."

Through the bars of the cell I saw Police Sergeant Trimmel—or, I should say, a shadow of Trimmel. He saw me at the same moment. He leaped off the iron cot, grabbed the bars and shook them. *"Du Schweinehund!"* he screamed. "It was you who did it!" He bared his teeth.

"What did I tell you," Hammer said matter-of-factly.

An hour or so later, after Trimmel had had a bath and shave and had dressed in his own clothes, we met in the *Dienstzimmer.* He was calm. "I realize it was not your fault, *Herr Doktor,*" he said after I had apologized. "Who could have known? The *Herr Oberst* behaved very reasonably during the train trip, explained the siege of the fortress of Przemyśl, even drew little diagrams on a piece of paper I gave him. We took a trolley to the hospital. I saw the name, and the kind of hospital it was written over the entrance, and he must have seen it too, but he didn't say anything, and so I had no warning at all. We waited in the *Herr Doktor*'s office. When the *Herr Doktor* came in, the *Herr Oberst* sprang to his feet, clicked his heels, and said, 'Herr Doktor, I deliver to you herewith the patient *Herr Doktor* Berczeller telephoned you about. Please, *Herr Doktor,* give me a receipt.' 'Bitte,' said *Herr Doktor* Hammer, 'und danke.' Here I got my breath back from the shock of hearing this. 'Wait!' I said. 'This is all wrong!' The *Herr Doktor* had scribbled a receipt and given it to the *Herr Oberst,* who clicked his heels and marched to the door. 'Come back!' I shouted, and stared after him, but the *Herr Doktor* put his arms around me in a special grip. 'Everything will be all right,' he said. I explained that the *Herr Oberst* was the patient and I was the police guard. 'I know, I know,' he said. 'In a few days you are going to feel perfectly wonderful.' 'Let me go!' I yelled, and twisted around and kicked him. Two big wardens rushed into the room, grabbed me, and carried me away.' "

"I am very, very sorry," Hammer said.

It is impossible to describe the look Trimmel gave him. Hammer rubbed his groin.

Needless to say, the *Herr Oberst* did not return to his chicken farm. His whereabouts remained a mystery for some time. Almost a year later I read a small item in the *Neue Freie Presse* about a white-haired man of distinguished appearance who had walked naked through the marketplace of a country town in the full glare of the midday sun.

❧ *XVI* ❧

FATHER KÖPPL AND
TIBERIUS CLAUDIUS

TIBERIUS CLAUDIUS VANAMIUS EQUES ALAE THRACUM.
TIBERIUS CLAUDIUS APLO EQUES ALAE EIUSDEM POSUIT.

Tiberius Claudius Vanamius,
horseman of a Thracian squadron, rests here.
Tiberius Claudius Aplo,
horseman of the same squadron, erected the stone.

On the stone was a portrait of Tiberius Claudius Vanamius, who
had been resting under it for almost two thousand years. The
stone was found in 1845 by an archaelogist digging on the outskirts of Mattersburg. Numerous discoveries followed, proving
beyond doubt that Roman legions had occupied all of Pannonia,
the district beyond the Danube, and had reached Mattersburg.
Their wives and families had followed. Typhoid fever was known
then, but not by that name; perhaps some had died of it—this
young woman, perhaps, with the gold wire around her teeth (a
Roman dentist had bound it there), and a string of blue beads
around her neck, a bracelet on her left arm, a bronze ring on a
finger of her right hand, a perfume bottle at her foot. I should

say, the places where her neck, her arm, her fingers, and her foot had been, for she was only a skeleton.

The excavations had led the diggers back into the deeper past, to the Stone Age. Fur-clad tribesmen had wandered and killed their prey where I drove my little Opel-Steyr, with Peter beside me on the front seat. This was ancient ground.

Father Köppl, the local priest, introduced me to Mattersburg's past. Over ninety per cent of the local population was Catholic. The church on the hill was early Gothic, but the interior was partly baroque, where the Tartars or the Turks or some other enemy had put it to the flames. A tall, strong man with round, shiny face, Father Köppl had many interests. Once, when we were talking about music, he mentioned the music of Roman times, which led to Tiberius Claudius Vanamius, who led to a recently published book, *Heimatkunde Mattersburg*, which Father Köppl gave me, an archaeologist's description of the town and environs. The priest and I had many chats in his study. How pleased he was one day, how his face shone, when he placed a few delicacies on the table for my inspection: remnants of an ax, half a dozen coins. Through a magnifying glass we studied the profile of Constantius II (337–361).

From Constantius II we jumped, in a manner of speaking, to Liszt.

"Did you know, *Herr Doktor*, that Franz Liszt was born in our Burgenland province?"

Yes, I was aware of it.

"Well," he continued with a humorous, twinkling look, "have you ever been in Raiding?"

This was the equivalent of asking a born-and-bred New Yorker, "Have you ever been to the top of the Empire State Building?" I had traveled many hundreds, even thousands, of miles but had never managed to get to the village of Raiding, ten kilometers away.

Feeling ashamed of myself, I drove there the following Saturday. I stopped to ask a villager for directions to the birthplace of Franz Liszt. He did not wait for me to ask but gave me the directions in an automatic voice. God knows how often he had done it.

The small house, with few rooms, was no different from its modest neighbors. Here a schoolteacher who was also a musician had given his son Franz piano lessons. In this dark room the little boy had touched the keys for the first time. Later on he was to be called "the greatest European."

Father Köppl, who, like most Austro-Hungarians, thought of Beethoven as the greatest musician of all, explained that without Liszt's encouragement and guidance Wagner would never have completed the Ring. "It was Max Reger, the composer, who said that he regarded Liszt's 'Faust Symphony' as Beethoven's Tenth. Do you agree, *Herr Doktor?*"

I said I did not agree, strongly.

"I too do not agree. But let us give our fellow countryman Liszt a chance." And out came the priest's archaic handwound portable phonograph, and we listened to the "Faust Symphony."

I was to spend many nights in that Gothic study, winding the phonograph, listening, talking, to return home after midnight with drowsy eyes and head full of Beethoven, Mozart, Bach, Haydn, Liszt, Brahms, and Roman coins, and Stone Age families huddled over the fire against the winter's saber-tooth cold, and a Thracian horseman who buried his dear friend and rode away to die, I suppose, in another land far from home.

After Frau Sonnenschein's death, her house stood empty for almost three years. She had been the last of one of the oldest Jewish families, and the property automatically became that of the Jewish community—a mixed blessing. The old baroque house, which had hardly been improved for centuries, was in an awful state, rather more a ruin than a habitable building. The Jewish Council considered leveling it. Many voices protested, quite rightly: the baroque exterior was one of the most beautiful in the ghetto. Well, then, the council would rebuild it, make it into a student dormitory.

Stonemasons, carpenters, painters arrived and set to work. I arrived, too. Enormous damage could have been done. Instead of hurrying off on calls, I interfered, gave directions: the fragile baroque designs must not be harmed; the tiny engravings mustn't be spoiled. The workmen looked at me with astonishment: it seemed the doctor was a nut after all. But I had a powerful ally in Aaron; when I finally departed to make my calls, he remained to supervise the work.

Finally the exterior was done and the workmen turned to the inside. What a mess! The house was a shambles: a few shaky tables and chairs, the bed where the old lady had died, a closet full of tattered clothes.

Aaron came galloping to the office. At the bottom of the closet the workmen had discovered a pile of papers, turned yellow and brittle, and a parchment scroll. "They were about to burn them! They still want to get rid of them! Come, exert your authority!"

I exerted my authority, such as it was, and the papers and the scroll were saved.

The papers were in Hebrew; Aaron said he would translate them. The parchment scroll, in Latin, I could make out. It was a marriage permit issued by the Duke of Esterházy, the lord of the land. I had heard about these permits but had never seen one. I took it to Eisenstadt, where there was a Jewish museum. Professor Csatkai, the custodian, told me it was priceless.

"What are you going to do with it?" he asked.

I explained that it was not mine. Back in Mattersburg I asked the *Herr Oberrabbiner.* "It seems you are a historian also," he said. "You discovered it—"

"I didn't discover it."

"Well, you saved it, which is better. So it is yours."

I returned to the museum with the news. There the scroll was

displayed as the donation of Herrn und Frau Dr. Richard Berczeller.

The *Herr Oberrabbiner* said that in the Community House
there were scores of old yellowed documents, untouched for centuries; perhaps I would like to go through them, screen them, see
what they amounted to. With Aaron's help I would, and did.

"The detective has now become a specialist in historical research," Maria remarked. "Where is the doctor I married?"

Aaron and I found that the Jewish community had been au-
tonomous until a century before. The birth-and-death register
dated from the fourteenth century; an inscription inside the temple gave the year 1362 as that of rebuilding and renovation. One
Torah roll had been purchased in 1435; another, a century later.
In the big book listing the meetings of the Community Council
there were gaps of two years, four years, sometimes ten and even
more. Each gap meant a tragedy: the Jews had been driven out of
the ghetto, which was itself severely limited in space: the original
grant had been no more than a hundred square yards. No wonder
the Jews added second and third stories to their dwellings; these
were not architectural refinements. Up was the only direction in
which they could go.

There was a document listing the seemingly endless "Jew
taxes," also called "taxes of tolerance": a tax on the temple, a tax
on ritual baths, a tax on the preparation of kosher meat, a tax on
the cemetery, taxes to pay for uniforms for the mighty Duke of
Esterházy's soldiers—and of course a tax on every kind of business, however humble. Even if the day's trade had brought in a
miserable penny or two, the penny or two was taxed.

Indeed these poor devils had great need of their religion and
their God.

"Aha!" said Aaron with a broad smile and waved a crisp old
yellow-edged page. "Our ancestors had other problems besides
taxes. Listen, my friend. This is a court report."

Slowly he translated: "Itzig and his wife, Chayeh, lived in mat-
rimonial harmony. A peddler, he left every Monday to sell his
goods and returned home on Friday, well before the Sabbath eve.
Their good friend Chaim ben Joshua, a distiller by trade, lived
next door. He was always helpful, would run errands and attend
to small business matters for Itzig during his absences.

"One day in the middle of the week Itzig did not feel well and
turned his steps toward home. He arrived shortly after midnight.
His wife was in bed where she belonged, but someone was in bed
with her. Who but Chaim ben Joshua, their good friend!

"Itzig demanded a divorce. He and his wife and their friend
stood in front of the rabbi. 'Can you swear on the Torah that
what you say is true?' the rabbi asked.

" 'I can, worshipful Rabbi,' Itzig replied.

" 'And you, Chaim,' said the rabbi, 'what do you have to say in
your defense, bearing in mind the Commandment that tells us
not to covet our neighbor's wife, to say nothing of getting into
bed with her?'

" 'I have this to say,' Chaim replied. 'My friend Itzig has told
the truth, but he does not understand it in the right way.'

" 'Can the truth be understood in more than one way?' asked
the rabbi.

" 'Yes, worshipful Rabbi,' Chaim replied, 'the right way and
the wrong way. I shall now demonstrate the right way. Yes, I was
in bed with my friend's wife, but I was there in a purely helpful
capacity. During the night in question I heard someone franti-
cally knocking on my door. I opened it and beheld my friend's
wife. She was much distressed, trembling indeed, because she had
heard mysterious noises in back of their house and was afraid evil
men were waiting to break in. She begged me to spend the night
in the house, sleeping in her absent husband's bed, while she, of
course, slept in her bed. Could I refuse my friend's wife in her
hour of need? I consented and went with her, and lay down in

Itzig's bed while she retired to her own. Suddenly we heard footsteps outside. With a scream of fear she jumped into my bed, or,
as I should say, Itzig's bed, and flung her arms around me. The
door opened. There stood Itzig. And that is the correct interper-
tation of the truth, worshipful Rabbi.'

" 'I see,' observed the rabbi and turned to Itzig's wife. 'Now,'
he said, 'please tell us the truth as you see it. What happened?'

" 'Worshipful Rabbi,' she replied, 'on that miserable night I
was lying in bed thinking of Itzig, my dear husband, far away,
when suddenly—' "

Aaron stopped. "Go on," I said.

He turned the page over, turned it back again, picked up another ancient page, glanced at it, put it down, picked up another
and another. "Damn it," he said, "wouldn't it be just my luck? I
can't find the rest!"

For a long time we continued with our task of screening the
yellowed old pages, but we were never to learn the truth according to Chayeh, wife of Itzig the peddler, who was found in bed
with her husband's best friend.

Our landlord, Herr Wilfing, was a man of thirty-five with thin-
ning blond hair and the benign eyes of a young calf. I was on the
very best of terms with him from the beginning, and so was Maria
with his wife. He belonged to the highest level of the local farmers and owned many prosperous acres, fruit orchards, vineyards,
and a fine two-story house with a wide courtyard, where oak and
linden trees grew. There were half a dozen rough tables and
benches there for Wilfing's friends, and he never stinted them,
bringing out jug after jug of wine. Even in his cups, I never heard
him quarrel with Frau Wilfing. They had only one sorrow in
their married life: she had given him two children, and they were
both girls. He badly wanted a boy.

"In my family," he told me, "there were ten children. I was the only boy. In my wife's family there were only girls. I should have thought of this before I married her. I am afraid we'll never have a boy, *Herr Doktor*."

"You must not give up, Herr Wilfing," I said. "You are young, and your wife is barely thirty. Keep on trying. One day you'll hit it."

His calf eyes looked sad. "Don't you have pills or a needle, something like that? I mean, I keep hearing that there is a cure for everything nowadays."

"As far as I know, there is nothing for that. Try."

Peter, of course, was Herr Wilfing's pet from the start. He would stand over the crib with doting calf eyes, and he rejoiced when Peter began to walk. Hand in hand, they walked here and there together, on short trips at first, then as far as Wilfing's orchards. Peter would sit with him on the driver's seat of his cart while the two girls sat in back.

Wilfing liked wine and drank not only his own from the big barrels in his cellar but also at the White Goose, the inn patronized by well-to-do farmers. He would return, walking not exactly in a straight line, holding on to Peter with one hand and with the other to his bigger girl, who in turn held the hand of her little sister. It often seemed to me that they were supporting him. Maria and I didn't worry; he wasn't really drunk, and we wanted Peter to know as much as possible of country life and country people. If we should ever move back to the city, he would have these memories. I suppressed my republican, anti-militaristic feelings when I heard him piping a martial song learned at the inn:

> *Mir san vow K. und K. Infanterie Regiment,*
> *Hoch und Deutschmeister.*

Heaven knows I enjoyed a few glasses with Herr Wilfing, and I recall with pleasure the long summer evenings in the courtyard when I played a popular Austrian card game, Preference, with him and a young judge of the local court. I can smell the hay in the stable and the leaves drenched by a summer shower; I can feel the lazy summer air and almost taste the wine. We were genuine card-players, deeply involved in the game, and sometimes hot words passed among us; but at the end all would be forgotten.

I returned home one evening to find Maria with a troubled brow. "Just look at Peter," she said.

Peter was in a state of hilarity. He had spent the afternoon with Herr Wilfing, and it was all too evident that they had stopped at the White Goose. Wilfing must have given him a little glass of wine, and another, and perhaps even a third. Peter sang with full strength the song *"Mir san vom K. und K. Infanterie Regiment, Hoch und Deutschmeister."* That was not all. He gesticulated and made deprecating gestures. "Those damn women," he said. "You screw them and screw them, and what comes out? Nothing but girls."

The next morning I spoke to Herr Wilfing. "Please be careful when the children are around, what you say to them. Last evening Peter said . . ." I repeated the words.

"Ah well," he said, clearly unconvinced. *"Manchmal muss man sich Luft machen.* You've got to let off steam once in a while."

But there were no more drinking sessions with biological comment for Peter.

For two years Maria had been the *Frau Doktor,* highly respected, her advice sought on medical and many other matters. She had learned to ignore the local anti-Semites and the snobs. Once a week she went to Vienna for postgraduate courses in the higher arts of cooking and baking, mostly baking. Far away were those formidable cakes that tasted like clay when they did not taste like candles. Mountains of Indianerkrapfen and Sachertorten filled the kitchen. I understood more than ever Goethe's "Nothing is harder to endure than a series of beautiful days." To tell the truth, I longed for simple, tasty *Hausmannskost*. But Maria was relentless in her scholarly fervor.

Around our house, on the main square, all the important events took place. The veterans' brass band blew; the non-Jewish fire department paraded, big men with solemn faces, marching in their gleaming boots and helmets and white gloves, followed by the engine. Funerals: again the band, blowing mournfully with deep oom-pahs, like grieving elephants. At the annual Corpus Christi procession the air smelled of incense and the starch of the little girls' lily-white dresses. Facing our window was a baroque Trinity column which had been put up by the happy survivors of a plague epidemic. During religious processions the priest always stepped down from under his canopy and knelt in front of the column. Something was always going on.

After the daily cleaning and tidying and looking after Peter and cooking and baking, Maria and our little maid, Anna, would stand together at the window to watch the passing show. Anna was twenty and very enthusiastic. The two of them would talk away and point out details and exclaim and laugh, or, if there happened to be a funeral, somberly comment on various features connected with the departed. Maria never lacked enthusiasm when she described these spectacles and events to me at the end of the day.

I remember very well a young peasant woman and her husband who came to my office on March 21, 1932, because that is Maria's birthday. Both of them had red handkerchiefs tied around their cheeks, and I assumed they had come for tooth-extraction. A country doctor also pulled teeth. In the old-fashioned way, which to my knowledge never did a bit of good, the sufferer always wrapped his head in a towel or handkerchief. For extraction without anesthesia I charged three schillings; for local anesthesia, five. Patients asked for tooth-pulling "with" or "without pain."

I was wrong. The young woman was badly bruised on her right cheek; her husband had a deep cut on his left cheek. They looked at each other with murderous eyes, and I did not ask questions—a marital quarrel, no rarity in my practice.

First I treated the woman by cutting away small pieces of excoriated skin and cleaning and dressing the wound. The man's cheek took five stitches, and I told him to come back in a week to have them removed. They did not thank me and leave; they stood there. "Well?" I said.

"It happened like this," the woman said. "This animal, my husband, came into the barn when I was feeding the pigs. '*Du Drecksau,*' he shouted. 'It's six o'clock already, and the pigs must be fed no later than five! They'll starve to death!' And with the handle of the hacksaw he was holding he hit me in the face, the son of a bitch."

"Yes, yes, very true," the man said fiercely. "I mean the part about the pigs. She always gets up late. But what about the rest of the story? Why so silent about that? Let me tell you why! When I came into the barn she was standing with her skirts raised. And standing with her was one of our young farmhands, with his fly open! Naturally I saw red and hit her. She grabbed the blade and carved up my face."

"Oh my God, what lies!" she shouted. "Sándor is a boy of sixteen! I could be his mother, almost! And doesn't a man open his fly for other reasons?"

"And at the same moment the woman lifts her skirts?" the husband inquired sarcastically. "Some mother! Quite a coincidence!"

"Why are you telling me all this?" I asked. "I'm sorry, but I have other people waiting."

"Why?" they said in unison. "Because we want a divorce!"

"Then you should go to a lawyer."

They stared at me with wide eyes. "A lawyer?" the woman said. "Why do you think we came here? Frau Wograndl from Pöttsching, she recommended you to us. The *Herr Doktor* is very good, very reliable, Frau Wograndl said."

Later I was to learn that a lawyer, Dr. Kellner (lawyers are called doctors in Germany and Austria), had occupied my office.

"What did *you* think," I asked, "when a lawyer treated your face and put the stitches into your husband's cheek?"

"Well—so?" the man said.

"Is stitching the cheek a lawyer's job?" I asked.

"A lawyer is a doctor, isn't he? Aren't you a doctor?"

"A physician!" I shouted. "A medical doctor!"

They considered this for a while. "Please go!" I said. "I told you, I have other patients!"

"What's the difference, after all?" the husband said stubbornly. "One doctor equals another doctor. Can't you take the case? I have confidence in you."

"I too," his wife said and gave me a coquettish smile.

Maria and Peter spent the hottest summer weeks of 1932 at Lake Balaton in Hungary, a paradise for children because the lake, the largest in Central Europe, is so shallow at the edge that one can walk almost a kilometer before the water is deep enough for swimming; it is thus also a paradise for mothers, for there is nothing to worry about. Siófok, the resort, was famous for elegantly dressed upper-middle-class ladies displaying the latest Parisian styles.

Lake Balaton is a hundred and fifty kilometers from Mattersburg, and Siófok is at the far, eastern shore of the lake—another fifty kilometers. On the atrocious roads, the trip took me five hours or more. One weekend it took a whole day, because I had no less than twelve flat tires. I arrived exhausted and irritable. But the next morning, when I swam with Peter holding on to my back, made the trip worth while. That night Maria and I danced to gypsy music, and she, "the Viennese lady," as she was called, had half a dozen young Budapest gallants begging for a dance.

On my way home I thought about them and experienced pangs of jealousy, which I can now confess, thirty-five years later.

I was alone with my practice, which in summer slowed down a great deal. I had time to read, time to go twice a week to Vienna for a course in electrocardiography and resume my acquaintance with that formidable machine. The interpretation of the tracings, which had to be developed in darkrooms, was still in its infancy. Four lead electrocardiograms were used instead of the twelve that are routine today; but from them one could diagnose myocardial damage—heart attacks—an enormous advance, which perhaps can be truly appreciated only by doctors who have lived through the period when absolute confirmation of a heart attack could be made only at the post mortem.

Karl Friedrich Wenckebach, who had done so much to develop electrocardiography, was no longer teaching. After his resignation as a teacher, he traveled to the Netherlands East Indies to study the effect of beri-beri, a nutritional disorder, on diseases of the heart. The course I took was given by one of his assistants. Patient after patient was put under the electrodes, from which wires led to the giant machine.

At this time I was called to the house of Herr Sagler, a well-to-do farmer in his fifties, a rather stout man who drank as much as anyone and smoked his pipe and worked in the fields fourteen hours a day. Perspiration was running down his face; he was dyspneic and complained about a crushing pain in his chest. I gave him a morphine injection. Ten minutes later the pale face was its normal ruddy color. *"Es geht scha besser, Herr Dokta,"* he said.

My clinical impression was, of course, a heart attack—but how could I prove it? I advised bed rest and said I would keep an eye on him.

In the kitchen I told Frau Sagler and the two grown sons that he was seriously ill. It would have been superfluous to advise hospitalization. I knew the answer in advance: People die in hospi-

tals; the surgeons cut them up, they perish, and are not even returned to the mourning family in one piece.

The next day my first call was to Herr Sagler. A wolfhound
came leaping toward me. I extended my doctor's bag; he sniffed it
and wagged his tail as though to say: Pass, friend. But no one else
was around. I went into the house, calling, "Frau Sagler?" No
answer. I knocked on the bedroom door. Silence. I opened it. The
bed was made. Herr Sagler was nowhere to be seen.

I looked out in the fields and saw the Sagler family at work. As
I walked toward them, Herr Sagler nodded his bushy white head.
"Sehens, Herr Dokta, I bin scha gesund!" he said jovially.

Oh, certainly, I could see that he was healthy! "I am taking you
home at once."

"But can't you see it? Look at me!"

"Am I the doctor or you?"

"I am healthy!"

"You are going to bed! If not, I wash my hands of you. Call
another doctor; see what he has to say."

"We have confidence in you, *Herr Dokta*," said the older son,
"but still, to put a healthy man to bed . . ."

"When there is work to be done," his father added.

"Listen," I said, "I propose a compromise. I will take Herr Sagler to Vienna. There we will make a picture of his heart. Then,
after looking at it, we will decide what to do next. Does this make
sense?"

They wished to know how I could take a picture of his heart
without cutting his chest open.

"That is not necessary. There is a machine with wires that does
all the work with no pain to the patient whatever."

Frau Sagler frowned but seemed to be convinced. "You promise
not to keep him in the hospital, *Herr Dokta?*"

"Yes, if the picture should not make it imperative."

"In God's name, then," Herr Sagler said, "let's go."

I drove him to Vienna. He looked well during the trip. I could not deny him his pipe. "There is nothing wrong with me," he said again and again, "but I did not want to offend you."

In the Vienna General Hospital the electrocardiogram showed the classic signs of damage to the anterior part of the heart; he had had a heart attack. It called for immediate hospitalization. I explained to him, ending with stern words: "You are ill, you are very ill. You must stay here. The heart picture has made it imperative."

He continued dressing. "I am going home. The machine does not know what I know."

I appealed to the other doctors present; they added their warnings, fuller explanations, and so on. Nothing helped. "Home," said Herr Sagler.

And so we traveled toward home, Herr Sagler beside me, smoking his pipe. There was no conversation. He was angry; I was angry; also I was despondent. I knew what I had seen. Half a dozen times I started to tell him again but a glance at his face told me: useless.

We were a little more than halfway to Mattersburg when I heard a little sound as though something had fallen to the floor. I looked at Herr Sagler. His mouth was wide open. The pipe lay at his feet. I stopped the car, took the stethoscope from my bag, opened his vest: no beat. He was dead.

As I drove on, the dead man beside me slumped down bit by bit, and he lay like a heap of old clothes when I drew up in front of his house. The wolfhound came running, suddenly stopped, sniffed the air, then raised his head and howled. I have never forgotten that almost instant recognition of death. It brought Frau Sagler and the two sons from the field where they had been working. The dog was still howling as the woman screamed.

There were five or six patients in my waiting-room—nothing serious. I said I was sorry, I could not see them that day. I felt sick. I lay down on the couch in the living room. Why had I come to this damned town? Why did I have to deal with stupidity, ignorance, pigheaded stubbornness? Anna, the maid, called that dinner was ready. I told her I had no appetite.

A few days later, after the funeral, which had been carried out with all the honors to which a war veteran was entitled, Frau Sagler and her sons, dressed in black, came to the office. "We wanted only to thank you," she said. "You did your best." The older son put three one-hundred-schilling notes on my desk.

Yet somehow I knew, I could read in their eyes the suspicion that would not die: If the doctor had not taken him to the hospital, would he not be alive today, working in the fields, drinking at the end of day, smoking his pipe?

⊰ *xvii* ⊱

TO GO OR TO STAY?

On August 30, Maria and Peter came back from Lake Balaton. Her first remark, "You're not looking well," was followed by a great bustling and noise of pots in the kitchen. *Gute Hausmanns-kost,* but also the inevitable Indianerkrapfen and Sachertorte.

The apartment, she said, was in a mess, not to mention my office. My desk could only be called an abomination. "But we will soon have things orderly and decent again," she concluded.

I was still feeling the shock of Herr Sagler's death on the seat beside me. After the apartment was, in Maria's words, orderly and decent again, I mentioned the tragedy to her. I felt I had to speak about it.

She understood that the experience had been a traumatic one but then tried to rationalize it. "Let me quote you for a change," she said. " 'Assassinations are the occupational hazard of kings.' This, I believe, came from Mussolini when he was still editor of a Socialist paper. Well, a doctor also has occupational hazards."

"How clever you are, Maria."

"Please," she said, "none of your irony."

"I mean it. It's good to have you home. But the way these coun-

try people behave—it's terrible, archaic. How stubborn they are
—utterly inflexible! How frustrated it makes you feel! Sometimes
I'm sick and tired of the whole thing."

"You chose to become a country doctor, didn't you?" Maria
asked. "Isn't that correct? Now just quiet down."

A letter arrived from the Krankenhaus der Stadt Wien.

Sehr geehrter Herr Kollege!

> Your leave of absence ends on December 1. You have had
> two extensions, as you know, and I am afraid that a third
> won't be possible. Professor Reiter, with whom I have dis-
> cussed your case, still considers you to be perfectly qualified
> to become an *Assistent* as soon as there is an opening. Please
> let me have your decision as soon as possible. Needless to say,
> we are all looking forward to seeing you again at the hospital.
>
>   With kindest regards,
>
>   Baumgarten

My first reaction was the same as when I'd received an exten-
sion, but then I realized that there could be no more; I would
have to decide once and for all. I read the letter again. Wasn't my
decision already made? I had a comfortable home, an excellent
office with modern equipment, all finally paid for after the seemingly interminable installments. Professionally I was satisfied
with my work; that is to say, I felt I had done as well as any
country doctor could, considering the stubborn nature of the patients, and so on. Would I exchange them for *city* people, who all
had their idiosyncrasies—many, many idiosyncracies? Another
most important consideration was that I was independent. How
would I feel in the hospital, with superiors watching me? Even as
a *Herr Assistent,* I would have the chief to reckon with. Not to
mention the post mortems—the satanic smile of Professor Erdheim if the clinicial diagnosis proved to be false, the piping voice:
"*Ja, Herr Kollege,* no pneumonia. A nice little cancer instead."

Maria read the letter. "I hope you will be sensible, Richard. The furniture—"

I felt irritated. "Kindly don't mention the furniture first! Anyway, it was shipped here from Vienna, can't it be shipped back? The first thing to consider is the philosophical aspect."

"Please," she said, "don't fall back on those big words of yours."

"I only mean that this is a decision for life."

"Now you change to pathos. It's all very simple, really. What you are offered now you could have had three years ago. *I* wanted to stay in Vienna, all your friends said you should stay there, and you were right on the verge of becoming an *Assistent*. And what did you say? How well I remember! You said, 'It's a dream. Let me dream a bit.' So! You made the dream a reality. And now that you're past thirty, you want to dream again?"

"Don't distort my words."

"I'm not distorting them. I am quoting you exactly. Let me quote my grandmother. When I told her I was breaking off my engagement to Ernst to marry you, she said, 'Beware of him, he's a dreamer.'" Maria looked at me. "Don't misunderstand," she said. "I don't regret it."

"You certainly shouldn't," I said. "Quite a dreamer, who works like a horse to take care of his family!"

"Every decent husband takes care of his family. Richard, I know you. Don't make a mistake you'll regret forever after."

There was no sense in continuing the discussion. I still had plenty of time to write that final letter—a letter of resignation.

September started with a burst of all kinds of illnesses and ailments, but mainly influenza. How many useless house calls I made! These people had no judgment whatever. For a sore throat I would drive for miles, come to the end of the road, and walk up a slippery path, muddy, full of potholes, in the rain. For pneumonia I would be called at the very last minute; the patient expired practically as I entered the door. I saw one dark, smelly sickroom after another and pursued the deadly routine work in the office: stitches and stitches and tooth-extractions "with" or "without pain."

After dinner I would settle down in the deep leather chair Maria had bought for my thirtieth birthday and read the morning paper, which had been brought from Vienna on the afternoon train. Often, far too often, I would doze off. I remember trying to read a novel by Annemarie Selinko about an ugly girl. It was readable but it put me to sleep. (Maria, a lightning-fast reader, told me the girl was not ugly at all.) One night in a half-doze I heard the chatter in the kitchen between Maria and our little maid, and the dishes and glasses, tink-tinkle; but at the same time I was not there, I was in the Krankenhaus der Stadt Wien—the tall buildings set among gardens, the clean rooms, the smell of cleanliness. Lo, I was in bed in my old hospital room under the good blanket with the Grecian frieze. Old Frau Feiglbauer in the thick eyeglasses was at the door. A gentle knock, a smile—I could see her toothless mouth. *"Herr Assistent,* time to get up." The Medical I Department—Sister Pia, marble-white face, pale blue eyes half closed behind silver-rimmed spectacles. She bowed a little to me—Sister Pia, bowing, just as she did to the chief! But then, I was the *Herr Assistent.* I made rounds, and she wrote my orders in the book she carried as if it were a prayer book.

Now suddenly I was no longer at the hospital; I was back in the house on the Parhammerplatz. Frau Tesarek—Gretl—came into the room, carrying a tray with frankfurters and chicken and cake and real coffee. I wasn't hungry. She wore wide skirts, like the peasant women. There was music in the room. I looked around and saw the tall window, the icicles outside. I breathed the frosty air, and adoringly I watched thin white fingers touch the yellowed keys.

A voice: "Look at you, falling asleep! Why don't you go to bed?" Maria was wearing the leaf-green embroidered apron she had bought in Siófok.

But I was wide awake, as one is after a little nap. "Are you tired?" I asked.

"No," she said. "Why? Do you want to talk a little?"

"I had a funny dream—sliding back into the past."

"I always said you had the talent to become a psychiatrist or an analyst. I still don't know the difference."

"They were unconscious wishes. I saw two girls I used to know, but in my dream each of them had your face."

"My faithful husband!"

"The only thing I know," I said, "is this: I'm all mixed up."

"And I know the reason. You are dead tired. You need a vacation. Why not take one?"

"What about my patients?"

"Call the City Hospital. A dozen young doctors will be delighted to substitute. They need the money."

"No," I said, "it wouldn't solve the problem. That letter's hanging over my head."

A call came from Ferdl, and I drove up the winding road. His youngest child, Franzl, had the measles. Ferdl's wife, Resl, was much relieved to hear the simple truth. "Those stupid women," Ferdl said. "For every *Schmarrn* they yell for the doctor. What about some target practice?"

I couldn't refuse. It was a foggy day in October; through the drifting gray I could see the fir-tree needles already covered in tiny flakes of snow.

The bulls'-eye seemed to skip aside every time I shot.

"No good today, *Herr Doktor*," Ferdl said. "You're thinking of something else."

"True," I said.

He put down his gun. "Then let's go to the cellar."

I sat down on a bench at the huge old table in the cellar while Ferdl picked up a kerosene lamp and walked away through the Gothic arch. His footsteps became fainter and fainter, and soon there was perfect silence. Then quiet little taps sounded in the distance—a little louder, louder, and the lamp came through the arch, and Ferdl was smiling at me and holding up a bottle.

"There are six cellars, one underneath the other," he explained. "The bottles in the lowest of all are reserved for special occasions, very special guests—an archduke, or something on that order." He uncorked the bottle. "The year of this—1806." The damp air immediately seemed to glow, to flower, to become spring. The wine he poured was liquid gold. Each glass became a giant golden pearl.

He lifted his. *"Prosit!"*

"Prosit!"

The liquid gold flowed down, and our stomachs rejoiced. We emptied the bottle.

"And so?" Ferdl said. "What's wrong, *Herr Doktor?*"

"My wife says I need a vacation. Personally I'm inclined to agree, but with a slightly different twist. I think I need to be somewhere off by myself."

"Sometimes the women are right," Ferdl said. "I have an idea. Up near the top of the mountain there's a hunting lodge, one of the duke's fancy notions. He thought of it, had the place built, then forgot about it. There's no electricity, only a well with clear, ice-cold water. There's a bedroom, another room with lots of books on the shelves. A few times a year I go up. It is silent as the mountain stones. How would it be if you went up there with supplies for a couple of weeks—candles, ammunition for your gun? No one would disturb you; even I wouldn't. How about it, *Herr Doktor?*"

"It sounds good. Let me think it over."

Maria gave the idea her approval: "Just the thing." I admit she astonished me; I had thought she would be against it and I would have to hold out sternly for this period of silence and meditation. "I'll pack a rucksack, bread, salami, butter, and eggs, also an alcohol burner and a nice little frying pan. I will show you how to make scrambled eggs; even you can do it, clumsy as you are when it comes to cooking."

In the hunting lodge I slept soundly, with no dreams. Sometimes there was the great silence of old stones and moss, as Ferdl had said; at other times a wind came down furiously from the icy sky and bent the trees below. There was a snowfall, and the world seemed to become smaller. It cleared, leaving the trees like white ladies in Empire gowns. I did some shooting, but more often I read, because I had discovered Voltaire's *Philosophical Dictionary* in the room with the books on the shelves. How had Voltaire found his way into the library of the arch-conservative Duke of Esterházy?

But I was still pondering the letter from the Krankenhaus der Stadt Wien.

A week later, Ferdl trudged up the mountain path with a bottle under his arm—1806, as before. "You look good," he said. "Your face is younger. But how do you feel?"

He asked in a delicate way, and I was moved. I told him about my dilemma as the wine flowed.

"I think I understand, *Herr Doktor*," he said at the end. "Now let me tell you *my* story. My father was a shepherd at Lackenbach, where the duke had some property—arable land, forests, ideal for hare-hunting. When I was sixteen, the proudest moment of my life came: I was assigned to carry the duke's gun. He was a poor shot, almost always missed. Once he told me to try. Well, I was lucky—of course, I also have a good eye. I didn't miss once. The duke gave me a job as assistant to the gamekeeper at Forchtenstein, a great honor. Soon the gamekeeper died, and I succeeded him—a terrific promotion at my age! I got married and we had two little girls, but my heart longed for Lackenbach, my childhood home with the garden and the blooming trees. My wife, may she rest in peace, listened to my complaints and said, 'But this is your home, a brick house, everything we could wish for. In Lackenbach what did you have? A thatched hut.'

"And still my heart longed for the old home.

"One day I could stand it no longer. I went to the duke and made my request. 'You are a fool,' he said, 'but since you won't be happy otherwise, all right, go and try it. I give you three months. Your position here will be kept open that long.'

"My wife wept bitterly at the joyful news—I mean, it was joyful for me. We packed our belongings and set off in the cart. How happy I was when I saw the old thatched hut, the garden, the blooming trees! This was my land, my home, this was my life!"

At this point Ferdl stopped and drank deeply.

"Little by little," he resumed, "I saw that matters had changed. Yes, the trees were in bloom, but the girls danced with boys I didn't know—young boys, almost children they seemed to me, strangers. I missed the fir trees, simple and straight and strong, and— But I can't express it. I told my wife, and she wept with joy. We packed the cart."

He drank again. *"Herr Doktor,* I think you should go back to Vienna and speak with the great professor who wrote to you. See for yourself. *Prosit!"*

I made an appointment with Dr. Baumgarten. I didn't sleep much the night of October 20, 1932. At six in the morning I left. I drove slowly; the appointment wasn't until ten. I got to Vienna at eight. What to do for two long hours? I remembered the Café Klinik. I hadn't been there since my graduation.

The Café Klinik had not changed. As always in the fall, the few outside chairs had been taken in. I smelled coffee and dust and tobacco. There was "my table" in the corner, with the view of the hospital morgue. No one was sitting there. I sat down and looked around and breathed in the familiar air and felt young again, and at home.

At the other tables students sipped their coffee and ate Gugel-hupf. Now from the kitchen came a short, heavy figure. He had not changed to speak of, either. He went from table to table, chatting with the students, calling them by their names. I waited impatiently for him to turn in my direction, for the beagle eyes to peer at me through the pince-nez. I waited for his surprise—*"Jessas, der Herr Doktor* Berczeller!"

He came to my table. His face was a question mark. "Your order?" he said.

"Don't you recognize me?" I asked.

He took off the pince-nez and wiped them and put them back in their proper place. He looked at me again and shook his head.

"Frau Tesarek," I said. "Liesl. Vera. Anny. Your gall bladder!"

"Hmmm," he murmured. "Let me think. In the meantime, your order?"

"Coffee and Gugelhupf—as always."

He left me. Soon he came back with a cup of coffee and a piece of Gugelhupf. But now under the white mustache there was the hint of a smile. "Thirty-eight years in the Café Klinik," he said. "Hundreds—no, thousands of customers, students who become doctors and go away. Other students come and sit at the same tables, thousands of them, as I said. But you I remember." He smiled broadly. "How could I forget? *Herr Doktor* Pick from St. Pölten! *Nicht wahr?*"

"Yes, Herr Franz."

I drank the coffee. I had no appetite for the Gugelhupf. I asked for the bill.

"One schilling and fifty."

I gave him two schilling bills.

"Danke, Herr Doktor Pick. *Auf Wiedersehen!"*

I telephoned the hospital and canceled the appointment. Then I walked out of the Café Klinik. It was drizzling, a typical late-October day in Vienna. I turned up my coat collar, got into my car, and stepped on the starter. The engine sprang to life. I drove down the road toward Mattersburg.

❧ *xviii* ❧

EPILOGUE: 1933

"Die Strasse frei für braune Bataillone . . ." The "Horst Wessel Song" sounded from the square. It was during my morning office hours, and my waiting-room was filled with patients. Still, I looked down on about three dozen youngsters in brown shirts marching in goosestep around the Trinity column, bellowing their song. For the first time, Nazis were marching in the streets of Mattersburg; no wonder, as Hitler's government ruled in neighboring Germany and was giving the weak Austrian Nazi movement encouragement.

Spring had started early in 1933, and the peasants were out working in the fields; only a few people stood on the sidewalks and observed the parade. The marching youngsters lifted their hands and shouted *"Heil Hitler!"* Soon the demonstration was over. One of my patients remarked that it was good that no local boy was among the marchers. "He would have gotten a good thrashing from his father," he said.

Soon after the demonstration ended, Aaron came to my office. He held a handkerchief to his forehead. When he removed the handkerchief, I saw a gaping wound.

"What happened?" I asked.

"The Nazis marched through the *Judengasse,* shouting, '*Juda verrecke.*' Hearing the commotion, I came out from my shop. I was outraged and raised my fists—"

"And they hit you?"

"No. In the excitement my spectacles fell from my nose; I groped around but couldn't find them, so I went back to my house and, blind as I am, I ran into a nail on the door."

I repaired the wound, putting in a few stitches. "You must be careful," I said.

"But think—Nazis in the *Judengasse,* shouting 'Death to the Jews'!"

"We still live in a democracy. Everybody is free to utter an opinion."

"Democracy, democracy," Aaron mumbled. "Do you have a few minutes' time?"

"Yes," I said. Aaron was the last patient of the morning.

"Now listen, *Herr Doktor,*" he said, "what are you doing still here? You have a wife and a little boy! And doctors are needed in Palestine, and if you don't like going there, go somewhere else. What we witnessed today was only the beginning. Anti-Semitism is a powder keg, and the Nazis have only to drop a spark into it to bring it to an explosion."

"Not here in Austria. Although Dolfuss is Chancellor, he is still no Hitler."

Aaron said, "Just look beyond the frontier. What happened to those twenty million Social Democrats and Communists? Leave while you can."

"And what about you?"

"I am an old man. Who needs an old printer? And you, as a doctor, must remember that an agoraphobiac won't cross the bridge. Never!" The railway station was beyond the bridge, on a hill.

It was lunchtime, and I walked over to our apartment.

"What happened?" Maria asked. "You look gloomy. I hope you're not upset about those stupid boys."

"I am not, really. The Nazis are not even sure of themselves in Germany."

"Then sit down and eat your lunch. Lately you're getting thin," Maria said.

My afternoon rounds began, as usual, in the *Judengasse*. One of the *Herr Oberrabbiner*'s children was ill. After the professional call was over, the rabbi invited me to his Gothic study. "What is your opinion, *Herr Doktor?*" He referred to the Nazi demonstration, which was the talk of the town.

I repeated what I had said to Maria.

"Right!" the rabbi said. "We must not lose the proper perspective. And may I add something? Do you recall Bismarck's saying after Prussia had defeated Austria in 1866? 'If Austria did not exist, it would have to be created.' That's what he said. What he meant was that a buffer state between the German and Slavic worlds was a historical necessity. And as far as we Jews are concerned, haven't we experienced trying times? The Almighty . . ."

While making calls in the hills, I met Ferdl.

"*Aba, Herr Dokta,*" Ferdl said, "too much fuss about nothing. And who cares what kind of government we have? They're all the same. We're small people. Maybe you know the story of the old, poor woman who queued up in front of a bakery during the short-lived Communist regime in Hungary in 1919. 'The world doesn't change,' the old woman sighed. 'In the old times rich people had it good; now it's the proletarians. But poor people stay always poor.'" Ferdl laughed over his joke. "I hope you're not worried about Hitler's Jewish program. I'm sure he doesn't mean it, but even if— It's still only a *program. Die Suppe wird nicht so heiss gegessen als sie gekocht wird.* The soup is not eaten as hot as it was cooked. But even if the program was carried out, who would do harm to *you?*"

After dinner I visited Father Köppl.

"As always, I agree with my illustrious colleague, the *Herr Oberrabbiner*," Father Köppl said. "May I add another historical fact? We clergymen like to quote from history. Once Austria was the leader of the 'Holy Roman Empire of German Nations.' But she was never an appendix of Germany, as Hitler wants her to become."

It was "our night." We scrutinized coins through the magnifying glass. We talked about Liszt, Paganini, Debussy, Berlioz. We listened to music. At midnight Father Köppl accompanied me to the winding staircase. He shook my hand warmly.

"Die Bäume wachsen nicht in den Himmel," he said reassuringly.

I walked home through the dark streets. I thought: It is to be hoped that the trees won't grow to heaven. I recalled the red flag with the mighty swastika which one of the Nazi boys had carried.

After the war I revisited Mattersburg. I walked through the *Judengasse,* framed by newly built houses. On the site of Aaron's house was a neat two-story building with geranium pots on the window sills. I thought of the Jews of Mattersburg who had been rounded up and driven to the railway station. I could see the men in their black suits, with beards; their women and children. And among them, a little old man with a helmet.

Aaron had crossed the bridge.